SUBSTANCE ABUSE TREATMENT
AND THE STAGES OF CHANGE

THE GUILFORD SUBSTANCE ABUSE SERIES
Howard T. Blane and Thomas R. Kosten, Editors

Recent Volumes

SUBSTANCE ABUSE TREATMENT AND THE STAGES OF CHANGE

Selecting and Planning Interventions

Gerard J. Connors
Dennis M. Donovan
Carlo C. DiClemente

Foreword by Barbara S. McCrady

THE GUILFORD PRESS
New York   London

© 2001 The Guilford Press
A Division of Guilford Publications, Inc.
72 Spring Street, New York, NY 10012
www.guilford.com

Printed in the United States of America

This book is printed on acid-free paper.

Last digit is print number: 9   8   7   6   5   4   3   2

Library of Congress Cataloging-in-Publication Data

Connors, Gerard Joseph.
   Substance abuse treatment and the stages of change : selecting and
planning interventions / Gerard J. Connors, Dennis M. Donovan,
Carlo C. DiClemente; foreword by Barbara S. McCrady.
      p. cm. (The Guilford substance abuse series)
   Includes bibliographical references and index.
   ISBN 1-57230-657-2 (hardcover)
      1. Teenagers—Drug use. 2. Substance abuse—Treatment. I. Donovan,
Dennis M. II. DiClemente, Carlo C. III. Title. IV. Series.

RJ506.D78 C66 2001
618.86′06—dc21   2001023248

To
Lana and Marissa
Anne, Collin, and Angelina
Lyn, Cara, and Anna

ABOUT THE AUTHORS

Gerard J. Connors, PhD, is Director of the Research Institute on Addictions at the State University of New York at Buffalo. He received his PhD from Vanderbilt University, and served on the faculty of the University of Texas Medical School at Houston before joining the Research Institute on Addictions as a senior research scientist. Dr. Connors's clinical research interests include treatment of substance use disorders, patient–treatment matching, early interventions with heavy drinkers, the role of the therapeutic alliance in addictions treatment, and treatment outcome evaluation. He is coauthor of the third edition of *Drug Use and Abuse*, and has authored or coauthored over 100 scientific articles and book chapters in the area of alcoholism and addictive behaviors.

Dennis M. Donovan, PhD, is Director of the University of Washington's Alcohol and Drug Abuse Institute, as well as Professor in the Department of Psychiatry and Behavioral Sciences and Adjunct Professor in the Department of Psychology at the University of Washington, where he also received his PhD. Before his appointment as Director of the Alcohol and Drug Abuse Institute, Dr. Donovan was affiliated with the Addiction Treatment Center at the Seattle Department of Veterans Affairs Medical Center, where he was involved in clinical, administrative, training, and research activities. He has over 120 publications in the area of alcoholism and addictive behaviors, with emphasis on social learning theory approaches to etiology, maintenance, and treatment; treatment entrance and engagement; evaluation of treatment process and outcome; relapse prevention; and patient–treatment matching.

Carlo C. DiClemente, PhD, is Professor and Chair of the Department of Psychology at the University of Maryland, Baltimore County. He received his PhD from the University of Rhode Island. Dr. DiClemente is the codeveloper, with Dr. James Prochaska, of the stages of change model. Over the past 20 years, Dr. DiClemente has authored numerous scientific articles, books, and book chapters examining the process of human behavior change and the application of this model in a variety of problem behaviors. He has been a faculty member at the University of Texas Medical School and the University of Houston, and has directed an outpatient alcoholism treatment program based on the stages of change model. Dr. DiClemente is coauthor of the self-help book *Changing for Good*, which is based on this model, and several professional books applying the model to addictive and health behaviors. His current research interests include alcoholism and substance abuse treatment, smoking initiation and cessation, dual diagnosis, the initiation of health protection, and health-threatening behaviors.

FOREWORD

What are the qualities and skills that make a substance abuse treatment provider effective? Research tells us that central qualities of the effective clinician are empathy, warmth, and positive regard, while developing and implementing a clearly articulated treatment plan and providing treatment for the problems that a client presents are important skills for the effective clinician. But putting these qualities and skills into action is a challenge. How *does* the individual clinician learn to express these central human qualities of caring and compassion with clients who often are difficult and unhappy about being in treatment, and whose central disorder often is characterized by behaviors that do not elicit empathy easily. And given the high prevalence of substance use disorders, and the incredible heterogeneity among clients, how *does* the clinician develop a thoughtful, individually tailored, and scientifically grounded treatment plan? *Substance Abuse Treatment and the Stages of Change* provides just such a framework, as well as a blueprint to help answer both of these questions.

First, the question of empathy. Developing genuine empathy for a client requires that the clinician be able to look beyond the client's behavior when using alcohol or drugs to understand the nature of substance use disorders and the difficulties inherent in changing what are often long-standing and pervasive patterns of thought and behavior. Drs. Connors, Donovan, and DiClemente provide clinicians with ways to perceive the alcohol or drug abuser that facilitates their feeling empathy for their client. They do so by describing the stages of change model, a model that makes understandable the difficulties that clients have in recognizing that they have a problem, in being ready to face and attempt to change that problem, and in dealing with challenges they encounter even when they decide they do want to change. Rather than feeling frustrated by or angry at a client who cannot "admit" a problem that is clearly evident to everyone around him or her, or discouraged by a client who fails to follow any of the clinician's suggestions for how to get sober, the clinician who truly understands the stages of change model can have an empathic and constructive inner dialogue: "Ah . . . this client is in precontemplation and doesn't recognize his problem . . . it must be difficult for him to have to come here . . . how can I support and empathize with his difficult position and still help him begin to realize how serious his problems are?" Or, "This client is still in the stage of contemplation . . . asking her to take active steps to change might drive her out of treatment . . . how can I help her be more ready to change?"

Nevertheless, understanding of a client's situation and accurate empathy about that situation are probably not enough for treatment to be successful—they must be combined with a good treatment plan. This is where *Substance Abuse Treatment and the Stages of Change* is unique among books about treating substance use disorders. The authors have gone far beyond the initial stages of change model by providing a useful blueprint for implementing treatment within the stages of change framework. The clinician will find clear guidance about how to assess the client's stage of change, how to plan and implement treatment in an individual or group setting with various populations with special treatment needs, and even how to apply the same framework to clinical work with families. The book is rich in clinical examples that bring the authors' ideas to life.

The book is strongly grounded in the scientific literature, and the authors have organized the research literature within the stages of change framework. Concepts and suggestions are well supported by empirical findings, but the authors have avoided the trap of slavish devotion to science. They are broad and nondoctrinaire in their ideas, and present ideas drawn from a range of theoretical and clinical perspectives (e.g., cognitive-behavioral, 12-step, and systemic). Science is the foundation upon which the book is built, but their creative flourishes make the final product unique and their own.

In the present era of accountability and efficiency in the delivery of health care, this book is timely and important. Clinicians who use the authors' framework and suggestions should provide treatment that is more efficient and effective because it will be well matched to the needs of their substance-abusing clients and delivered with the warmth and empathy that are crucial to work with this population.

As a reader, you have made a wise choice in selecting this book. You will learn a way to think about substance-abusing clients and new strategies, as well as how to select more effectively from the armamentarium of treatment strategies you already know. You won't find a "how-to-do" manual in the pages that follow; rather, you will find a "how-to-think" book. And if you can incorporate these new ways of thinking into your clinical work, you and your clients will be richly rewarded.

BARBARA S. MCCRADY, PHD
Rutgers—The State University
of New Jersey

PREFACE

Treatment for alcohol and drug use disorders has become a major part of mental health services in recent years. As part of this trend, professionals with a range of experiences and training, including alcohol and drug counselors, psychologists, social workers, and psychiatrists, have been involved in treating people with substance abuse disorders and their families. In addition to the wide range of treatment providers, a variety of treatment techniques and interventions are used. While there is advantage in this diversity in providers and treatment, integrating information about treatment and communicating it to all of the service providers who want it can be difficult, at best. This book was conceived and written to reach the wide range of clinicians who treat substance use disorders. Throughout this book two issues remain fundamental. The first concerns the client's receptiveness or readiness to use different methods of change, and the second concerns what constitutes those methods.

These issues are addressed in this volume through application of the stages of change model. The model offers an integrative framework for conceptualizing and implementing behavior change among substance abusers. Indeed, the stages of change model has emerged over the past decade as one of the most visible, popular, and influential models in the addictions field, and the concepts introduced by the stages of change model have become part of the lexicon of substance abuse treatment providers.

Lacking, however, have been efforts to integrate the present themes with treatment interventions and to provide a vehicle for the application of the stages of change model to the treatment of substance use disorders. This volume is intended to address that void.

It is our hope that, taken together, these efforts will benefit clinicians in their continuing efforts with clients suffering from substance use disorders.

ACKNOWLEDGMENTS

This book could not have been conceived and developed without the support and assistance of a number of people. We are indebted to Stephen A. Maisto for his seminal contributions in the developmental phases of the project. Julianne Pawlik, Mark Duerr, and Beverly Artis provided patient and expert assistance in the preparation of the manuscript. We thank Howard T. Blane for his support and guidance, and Jim Nageotte, our editor at The Guilford Press, for his editorial expertise. Finally, we would like to thank our families for the support and encouragement they provided throughout this endeavor.

CONTENTS

1

BACKGROUND
AND OVERVIEW

Alcohol and drug use[1] is a common occurrence in today's society, with such use often associated with a variety of medical, psychological, and social problems (Frances & Miller, 1991). As we discuss later in this chapter, the financial costs to society are extremely high, and the human suffering is considerable. For these reasons society has looked to treatment as one way to modify an individual's substance use and its concomitant problems.

This book is a practical guide to treatment of alcohol and drug use disorders in adults that is based on the most current theory and research. We devote this chapter, as a foundation, to highlighting the prevalence of drug use and the consequences of harmful drug use. We then discuss efforts to formally define patterns of alcohol and drug use that are identified with people who participate in self-help or professional treatment programs. Following that, we note that treatment has been given a lot of attention in the alcohol and drug fields because of the urgency felt to change alcohol and drug use patterns that are harmful to individuals, society, or both. Accordingly, we then introduce the stages of change model, a conceptual approach to behavior change that has had a significant impact on the treatment of substance abusers and is used as a focal point for crystallizing the diverse information presented in this volume.

ALCOHOL AND DRUG USE

The emphasis of this book is on alcohol and drug use that results in problems in functioning. A step toward understanding such drug use patterns is to view an individual's use in the context of drug use in society in general. Along these lines, the national surveys of alcohol and other drug use that have been taken periodically over the past several decades are instructive.[2]

In the 1997 National Institute on Drug Abuse (NIDA) survey (U.S. Department of Health and Human Services, 1998), a variety of data about adult drug use in the United States were collected. These data include overall prevalence of use during the past year and past month for different drugs, including alcohol and tobacco cigarettes. In this case, "use" means the respondent used the drug in question at least once during the time period in question. Several findings stand out. First, alcohol (used by 64% in the past year) leads the use list, followed by cigarettes (used by 33%) in a distant second place. Marijuana and hashish (at 9%) head the list of illicit drug use. These relationships hold up both for use in the past year and for use in the past month.

The prevalence of drug use differs with characteristics of people. For example, the prevalence of drug use in the past month varies as a function of age. Individuals in the age range 18–25 have the highest prevalence of use of cigarettes (used by 41% in the past month) and of any illicit drug (used by 15%). Rates of alcohol use in the past month were highest among participants in the 26–34 age group (used by 60%).

Substance use during the past month also varies according to ethnic/racial group and gender. The most striking findings are the gender differences. Men (at 7%) were twice as likely as women to report use of marijuana in the past month and considerably more likely than women to report any alcohol use (58% vs. 45%). For ethnic/racial differences, whites (at 55%) more frequently reported any alcohol use than did Hispanics (42%), blacks (40%), and those of another ethnicity/race (37%), but blacks (at 6%) reported marijuana use slightly more frequently than did the other three groups (5% for whites, 4% for Hispanics, and 5% for those of another ethnicity/race).

The national survey data provide clinicians with the best single frame of reference to evaluate and interpret substance use by their clients.[3] The quality of the interpretation tends to improve with attention to subgroup differences. That is, any given client's pattern of substance use can best be viewed in the context of what is typical for his or her subgroup as defined by characteristics such as age or gender. Of course, this principle might be applied to a range of sociodemographic (e.g., years of education) and other characteristics of the person. Importantly, knowledge of the norms of substance use for a client's subgroup also helps the clinician and client to plan treatment goals and to anticipate the likely obstacles and supports in achieving and maintaining them.

THE PRICE OF DRUG USE

The consequences of alcohol and drug abuse are costly. "Cost-of-illness" studies provide a detailed estimate of the cost, in dollars, of a given illness or disease. A major cost-of-illness study on alcohol and drug abuse was prepared by Harwood, Fountain, and Livermore (1998). Using detailed data for 1992, these researchers estimated that the economic cost to U.S. society alone from alcohol and drug abuse was $246 billion ($148 billion for alcohol abuse and alcoholism and $98 billion for drug abuse and dependence). The estimate for alcohol was similar to those calculated over the past 20 years (when adjusted for inflation and population growth), while the estimates for drugs over that period have demonstrated a steady and strong pattern of cost increases. These costs were distributed primarily among direct treatment and other health care expenditures, the value of reduced or lost productivity due to impairment on the job, and the value of productivity lost due to premature death. Other costs included those related to crime (e.g., lost property), motor vehicle crashes, fires, and the value of lost productivity of victims of crime, incarcerated convicts, and caregivers (Rice, Kelman, Miller, & Dunmeyer, 1990, p. 5).

The estimated costs of alcohol and other drug abuse in 1992 were staggering. By applying the same model and computations, researchers estimated that the costs of alcohol and drug abuse in 1995 climbed to $166.5 billion and $109.8 billion, respectively (Harwood et al., 1998). Cost-of-illness studies are recognized as imprecise. Still, such research brings home the striking level of consequences we are addressing in alcohol and drug treatment. And cost-of-illness studies do not at all touch the cost in human suffering related to substance abuse.

A BRIEF INTRODUCTION TO TREATMENT

As with many of the other concepts in this field, treatment has been variously defined. We use the definition arrived at by consensus in the Rinaldi et al. (1988) Delphi Survey study. According to that study, treatment was agreed to be an "application of planned procedures to identify and change patterns of behavior that are maladaptive, destructive, or health injuring; or to restore appropriate levels of physical, psychological, or social functioning" (Rinaldi, Steindler, Wilford, & Goodwin, 1988, p. 557).

With this definition, it is easy to imagine many different procedures that could be called treatment. The procedures that are used in the treatment of the substance use disorders can be broadly classified into individual treatment, marital/couple/family treatment, and group treatment. We discuss each of these modalities in detail in subsequent chapters. Note that the major modes of treatment are practiced in different settings, including inpatient/residential, partial hospital, and outpatient.

STAGES OF CHANGE MODEL

A person's resistance to a given treatment effort has been a long-standing and sometimes frustrating problem for clinicians. In particular, individuals who present for treatment of substance use disorders have the reputation among clinicians of being unduly resistant or unwilling to change. Therefore, it would be useful to have a model or theory that would help to address the problem of how to match an individual's treatment to his or her commitment to change. One way to achieve this end would be to have a chart of the course of change in general and then to coordinate the treatment procedure that best fits where the person is in the course of change. Such a chart would be descriptive of a model of change.

In fact, several stages of change models have appeared in psychotherapy literature over the years (e.g., Horn, 1976; Kanfer, 1986; Rosen & Shipley, 1983). We have chosen to use the Prochaska and DiClemente (1982, 1984, 1992) "stages of change" model as our preferred way of addressing a person's readiness for change. This stages of change model was developed from research on the treatment procedures or techniques that people use in modifying a particular problem behavior. We have selected this model from among the other possibilities for two reasons. It has generated more research than other models, and much of that research has pertained to people trying to change their patterns of substance use. Moreover, this research has provided evidence for the validity of the stage of change construct and for its clinical utility (e.g., Carney & Kivlahan, 1995; Heather, Rollnick, & Bell, 1993; Willoughby & Edens, 1996).

During the past 15 years or so the stages of change model itself has undergone changes to some degree, mainly as a result of the now fairly extensive research findings on the model that have been published. However, the changes in the model relate more to content than to underlying concept so that the ideas that originally generated the model remain largely intact. The most current detailed versions of the model are presented by Prochaska and DiClemente (1992) and DiClemente and Prochaska (1998).

The current model posits five stages of change, called, from earliest to latest, precontemplation, contemplation, preparation, action, and maintenance.[4] People who are in the precontemplation stage show no evidence of intent to change a problem behavior. They may be unaware that their behavior is a problem, or aware that it might be but unwilling to do anything about it, or may be discouraged about changing the behavior as a result of past failed attempts to do so. The precontemplator tends to see the behavior as having more positives than negatives for him or her and therefore judges that the behavior is under control or at least manageable.

During the contemplation stage of some problem behavior, individuals are considering changing it. Thoughts about change might include the specific personal implications of the problem and what the consequences of change might entail. Contemplators are more visibly distressed about their problem behaviors than are the precontemplators and have begun to weigh the positives and negatives of change. They also search for information relevant to the problem behavior.

The preparation stage covers people who are ready to change in both attitude and behavior. These individuals intend to change soon and have incorporated their experiences of previous tries at change. As noted in DiClemente et al. (1991), people in the preparation stage may have begun to increase self-regulation and to change the problem behavior.

When people are in the action stage, behavior change clearly has begun. Accordingly, individuals in the action stage need skills to implement specific behavior change methods. They also need to be aware of various psychological (cognitive, behavioral, emotional) events that may work against their efforts at behavior change. Furthermore, there is a need to learn ways to prevent major reversals, such as an abstinent alcoholic taking a drink and returning to prechange patterns and levels of alcohol use. Such skills are essential to maintaining the desired change in a problem behavior and are especially important in changing alcohol and drug use disorders. According to Prochaska and DiClemente (1992), the action stage lasts an average of about 6 months in people working to change their substance use.

The last major stage of change is maintenance. When in this stage, individuals sustain and strengthen any changes they have made in the problem behavior. In this regard, such changes, even after 6 months, may not be well established and may take a few years to be "secure."

We should pause here to highlight several fundamental points about the stages of change. First, as may have been clear in our presentation of the stages, the stages describe attitudes, intentions, and behaviors about change (Prochaska & DiClemente, 1992). Second, the "change" sought after is in a specific target behavior, such as alcohol use or cocaine use. That is, commitment to change one behavior, such as alcohol use, may say nothing about commitment to change another, such as cigarette smoking. Third, the model is used to describe voluntary change processes rather than mandatory or coerced change, in which the individual has no options regarding his or her problem behavior. Moreover, the model is assumed to apply to efforts to change with or without the help of formal treatment. And lastly, each stage refers to a time period and to tasks one must complete before moving to the next stage. People may differ in the amount of time they spend in a stage, but the activities and processes involved to progress from one stage to the next one are similar for everyone.

Table 1.1 summarizes each of the stages of change and the features associated with it. Interventions that are most effective in each stage are a major topic of this book and of ongoing research projects by a number of investigators. For precontemplation, we have noted a "negative" intervention in that we suggest what *not* to do. Clearly the field needs to do more research on increasing the commitment to change in individuals who do not see they have a problem that is causing themselves or others distress.

TABLE 1.1. Stages of Change and Associated Features

Stage of change	Main characteristics of individuals in this stage	Intervention match	To move to next stage
Precontemplation	• No intent to change • Problem behavior seen as having more pros than cons	• Do *not* focus on behavioral change • Use motivational strategies	• Acknowledge problem • Increase awareness of negatives of problem • Evaluate self-regulatory activities
Contemplation	• Thinking about changing • Seeking information about problem • Evaluating pros and cons of change • Not prepared to change yet	• Consciousness raising • Self-reevaluation • Environmental reevaluation	• Make decision to act • Engage in preliminary action
Preparation	• Ready to change in attitude and behavior • May have begun to increase self-regulation and to change	• Same as contemplation • Increase commitment or self-liberation	• Set goals and priorities to achieve change • Develop change plan
Action	• Modifying the problem behavior • Learning skills to prevent reversal to full return to problem behavior	• Methods of overt behavior change • Behavioral change processes	• Apply behavior change methods for average of 6 months • Increase self-efficacy to perform the behavior change
Maintenance	• Sustaining changes that have been accomplished	• Methods of overt behavior change continued	

Note. Data from Prochaska and DiClemente (1983, 1992).

In the alcohol and drug treatment field such lack of awareness is commonly referred to as "denial" (a topic addressed in greater detail in Chapter 2). While imposing behavioral change methods is not as likely to be as effective with precontemplators as with those at other stages, a variety of verbal persuasion techniques, such as motivational interviewing (Miller & Rollnick, 1991), do hold considerable potential for helping clients advance to the contemplation stage.

Consciousness raising simply refers to learning more about a problem—the individual in the contemplation stage exposes himself or herself to what information is available. This contrasts with the behavior of the precontemplator, who tends to avoid facing anything related to a problem. Self-reevaluation similarly is looking at oneself as a way of gathering information or consciousness raising. The person asks the question, for example, How does cigarette smoking or getting drunk make me feel about myself? (Prochaska & DiClemente, 1983). Environmental reevaluation entails reviewing how the problem in question affects the people and situations in the person's life space.

Note that at the earlier stages of change overt behavior change methods are not the best match for the person. Better timing for such methods would be when the individual is in the action and maintenance stages, although there may be some initial use of behavior change methods in the preparation stage. Examples of these initial methods are varied and include use of a helping relationship, counterconditioning, reinforcement management, and stimulus control (Prochaska & DiClemente, 1983).

The last column heading of Table 1.1 summarizes what has to happen for a person to progress to the next stage of change. As we noted, the model assumes that these events must occur for progress to be made. Presumably the interventions in the final column of the table would help a person to accomplish the requisite tasks for progression to the next stage of change.

Although we describe these stages and a person's progress through them as linear (one stage leads to the next), in practice people commonly cycle back from an advanced stage to an earlier one. The stages of change model is a cyclic model—that is, individuals may go back to earlier stages of change after reaching a later one. This may happen a number of times before the person makes it to the maintenance stage for good. In the addictions, cycling is normative—individuals often "successfully" change a problem numerous times before the change is stable (Brownell, Marlatt,

Lichtenstein, & Wilson, 1986). Mark Twain's comment that "Quitting smoking is easy—I've done it many times" is apt. In Chapter 9 we expand the stage of maintenance to include the critical topic of relapse. Although conceptually an individual could relapse while still in the action stage, the problem of relapse traditionally has been thought of and discussed most in the context of maintenance of change.

An excellent illustration of the typical course people take in changing addictive behavior was presented by Prochaska, DiClemente, and Norcross (1992) and is reproduced here in Figure 1.1. The spiral model reflects the time-tested observation that the course of change is not linear.

The spiral model reflects another critical facet of change that gives hope to changers and clinicians alike. Even though a person may work to a later stage of change but reexperience problems that send him or her back to an earlier one, in most cases the person does not go all the way back to the precontemplation stage. Instead, he or she typically reverts to the contemplation or preparation stage for varying periods of time before advancing again. And often something is learned from a relapse so that the person does not fall all the way back to the spiral's entrance, but in-

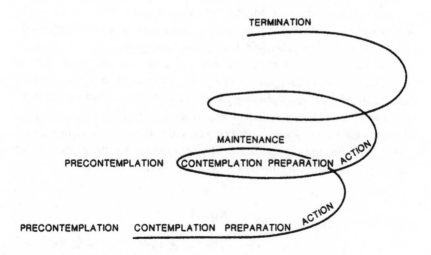

FIGURE 1.1. A spiral model of the stages of change. From Prochaska, DiClemente, and Norcross (1992, p. 1104). Copyright 1992 by the American Psychological Association. Reprinted by permission.

stead to some higher level on the spiral. Of course, the challenge is to get people out of the cycle of advance–revert–advance and into the top exit of the spiral, called termination in Figure 1.1—the point at which the person feels secure in his or her maintenance of change.

The stages of change model presents an excellent way to organize the vast amount of information that is available on treatment of substance use disorders. The model is based on clinical research and has important implications for clinical practice. We elaborate on these implications throughout this volume.

SUMMARY

• Alcohol and drug use are common among the general population. Use varies with several social and demographic variables, such as age, gender, and race.

• The effects of alcohol and other drug use cost society staggering sums of money and impose enormous human suffering on millions of individuals.

• Treatment has been defined in many ways. In this volume, we use the definition set forth by Rinaldi et al. (1988), namely, the "application of planned procedures to identify and change patterns of behavior that are maladaptive, destructive, or health injuring; or to restore appropriate levels of physical, psychological, or social functioning."

• The content of treatment and a person's receptiveness to it are fundamental to behavioral change. This volume utilizes the stages of change model to conceptualize the process of change and as a basis for deriving treatment content and implementing it. The stages of change model includes five stages, called precontemplation, contemplation, preparation, action, and maintenance. The termination of this process occurs when the person is secure in his or her maintenance of change.

NOTES

1. In this volume we use the terms "alcohol and drugs" or "drugs" as mutually *inclusive* terms. In fact, to say "alcohol and drugs" is redundant, since alcohol *is* a drug. However, because of the ways in which reports of basic and clinical research and other literature in the field have been written or organized, we will at times distinguish between alcohol and other drugs. We also should note that

alcohol and other drugs typically are talked about by the population in general as though they are distinctly different.

2. For this discussion we use data presented by the National Institute on Drug Abuse (NIDA) from its 1997 national household survey (U.S. Department of Health and Human Services, 1998). In this survey, interviews were completed by 24,505 respondents. Although the sample did include persons living in places like shelters, rooming houses, and college dorms, it did not include those who were in jail or military personnel. Overall, the national household surveys provide the best single description of frequency and quantity of different drug use among adults in U.S. society.

3. In the treatment of substance use disorders there is inconsistency among professionals in their use of the words "patient" or "client" to refer to individuals presenting for treatment. Often the term chosen depends on the treatment setting—that is, individuals in hospital inpatient settings are more likely to be referred to as patients while persons receiving treatment in outpatient community clinics are more likely to be referred to as clients. In this volume we use the terms "patient" and "client" as synonymous to refer to an individual who is in formal treatment for his or her substance use problems.

4. This discussion draws heavily on a chapter by Prochaska and DiClemente (1992). The stages presented are but one component of a broader transtheoretical model of behavior change (Prochaska, 1984; Prochaska & DiClemente, 1982) that also addresses levels of change and the process of change, components of which are discussed as appropriate in other sections of this volume.

┌─────┐
│ 2 │
└─────┘

THE STAGES OF CHANGE

Chapter 1 provided an overview of the stages of change model. In this chapter we discuss each of the stages of change in greater detail. As part of our description of these stages, we present and analyze clinical scenarios. These case scenarios are intended to illustrate, from a stages of change perspective, what clinicians may expect from individuals who present for evaluation or treatment with a substance use disorder.

Following this, we shift our attention to some general clinical issues relevant to the respective stages of change. In terms of the precontemplation, contemplation, and preparation stages of change, we focus in particular on the concepts of denial and resistance. These concepts are pertinent to the precontemplation, contemplation, and sometimes the preparation stages because they are commonly viewed in the field as crucial to the processes of taking initial steps to address a problem. Traditional perspectives on denial and resistance are reviewed and their presumed relationship to treatment outcome discussed. This is followed by a presentation on some recent reformulations of denial and resistance. Particular emphasis is placed on motivational techniques and their relevance to the treatment of clients with substance use disorders. Finally, we address as well some of the clinical issues that arise in working with clients in the action and maintenance stages.

THE PRECONTEMPLATION STAGE

As implied by the term, individuals in the precontemplation stage are either unaware or ignorant of their alcohol or drug use problem, or if aware are not thinking seriously about making changes in their substance use. Prochaska and DiClemente (1984) have offered several factors that can contribute to a person's being a precontemplator. One is that such individuals tend to be uninformed about the effects of their substance use on themselves or on others. An example would be the alcohol or marijuana abuser who in a solitary manner engages in heavy use but is unaware of potential long-term negative effects of such use, such as respiratory disorders.

Although some substance abusers are unaware of the dangers associated with their drug use, others, according to Prochaska and DiClemente (1984), simply are not receptive to indications that their alcohol or drug use is a problem. Such an attitude frequently has been conceptualized as denial or resistance, which is discussed in greater detail later in this chapter. The precontemplation stage can describe individuals who seek clinical services but who do so solely to placate others and not really to make changes in their alcohol or drug use (McConnaughy, DiClemente, Prochaska, & Velicer, 1989; Prochaska & DiClemente, 1984). Some characteristics of precontemplators are listed in Table 2.1.

Much of the early research on the stages of change model was conducted with smokers, many of whom would meet the criteria for nicotine dependence (American Psychiatric Association, 1994). In one study DiClemente et al. (1991) reported on the characteristics of smokers vol-

TABLE 2.1. Common Characteristics of Individuals in the Precontemplation Stage

Defensive

Resistant to suggestion of problems associated with their drug use

Uncommitted to or passive in treatment

Consciously or unconsciously avoiding steps to change their behavior

Lacking awareness of a problem

Often pressured by others to seek treatment

Feeling coerced and "put upon" by significant others

Note. Adapted in part from Prochaska and DiClemente (1983, 1984).

unteering for a smoking cessation program involving brief interventions. As part of the study, precontemplators were compared to contemplators and persons prepared for action-taking. For the purposes of this study, precontemplators were defined as smokers who were not giving serious consideration to stopping smoking during the upcoming 6-month period. DiClemente et al. (1991) found that precontemplators, relative to contemplators and subjects ready to change, reported fewer previous attempts at quitting, fewer concerns about quitting, more temptations to smoke, less confidence about quitting, and more advantages and fewer disadvantages of smoking. Precontemplators also used fewer activities related to smoking cessation (e.g., consciousness raising, self-evaluation, counterconditioning). Not surprisingly, and supportive of the stages of change model, the precontemplators made fewer attempts at quitting than did the other participants.

The precontemplation stage also has been studied among alcohol abusers. DiClemente and Hughes (1990) assessed stages of change with a large group of adults initiating outpatient alcoholism treatment. The clients were assessed not to be in need of detoxification or of an extended inpatient treatment regimen. They all completed a questionnaire, the University of Rhode Island Change Assessment Scale (URICA), that measures stages of change (see Chapter 3). Based on their responses to the questionnaire items, these clients fell into one of five "profiles" based on patterns of scores reflecting precontemplation, contemplation, action, and maintenance. The profiles were labeled precontemplation, ambivalent, participation, uninvolved, and contemplation. Two of these groups have relevance to our understanding of precontemplators. The first included clients labeled simply as being in precontemplation. These clients scored above average on the precontemplation scale and below average on the contemplation, action, and maintenance scales. As such, these are individuals who do not view themselves as having a problem with alcohol, are not contemplating change, and are not taking steps to effect changes in their drinking. According to DiClemente and Hughes (1990), the clients in this precontemplation group reported lower levels of concern about their alcohol use and lower scores on two alcoholism scales (general alcoholism and alcoholic deterioration) of the Alcohol Use Inventory (Horn, Wanberg, & Foster, 1987) relative to clients falling into groups characterized by more contemplation and action regarding their alcohol use.

Nevertheless, the precontemplators' level of drinking was comparable to that of clients thinking about changing or already initiating change, and their reported levels of withdrawal symptoms were also comparable.

The precontemplation cluster has been replicated by Carney and Kivlahan (1995) in their study of over 400 male polydrug users entering addictions treatment at a veterans hospital. Using a clustering procedure to study these clients' responses on the URICA measure, Carney and Kivlahan (1995) identified a group of polydrug users who were high on the precontemplation scale and low on the contemplation, action, and maintenance scales. Thus, a population of precontemplators is readily identifiable across alcohol and other drug abusers.

We noted earlier that being in precontemplation does not preclude entry to treatment for a substance use disorder, although generally the person does not acknowledge a problem and is arriving mainly to placate others. This would appear to be the case for the precontemplators identified by DiClemente and Hughes (1990) and by Carney and Kivlahan (1995), all of whom were nevertheless seeking admission to addictions treatment programs.

Another cluster of individuals identified by DiClemente and Hughes (1990) was labeled ambivalent. The ambivalent clients scored particularly high on the precontemplation scale (higher than the clients in the precontemplation cluster described earlier) but also above average on the contemplation, action, and maintenance stages. As such, this is a seemingly paradoxical group. On the one hand, they are predominantly characterized by precontemplative attributes. On the other hand, they also are above average on contemplation and action attributes. Given this pattern of apparent conflict, DiClemente and Hughes (1990) have characterized this cluster of clients as "somewhat reluctant or ambivalent about changing their alcohol-problemed behavior" (p. 223). Although high in precontemplation, they appear to be closer to contemplating change than the clients in the precontemplation group. This pattern of scores on the URICA scales also was found in a subgroup of the polydrug users studied by Carney and Kivlahan (1995).

Taken together, precontemplators are individuals who are unaware or resist becoming aware of their substance use problem. Ironically, they do appear frequently at treatment settings—but usually in response to external pressures such as family, job, or legal ultimatums.

Case Example of a Client in the Precontemplation Stage

Sam W is a 28-year-old married man who was seen at an outpatient drug treatment program for an intake evaluation. This initial appointment was scheduled by his wife Joan, who had indicated to the telephone reception-ist that Sam's use of crack cocaine was out of control and that he needed treatment.

Sam appeared 15 minutes late for his intake evaluation. He was wearing slacks and a sports shirt and was well groomed. His wife accom-panied him, but she preferred to wait for him in the waiting room and did not participate in the session. Sam began the session by stating "for the record" that he was not experiencing any problems associated with his drug use and that his wife was simply being narrow-minded and at-tempting to control him. He admitted that he was using marijuana and crack cocaine, but he asserted that both were being used recreationally and nonproblematically.

He described his marijuana use first. He had started smoking in high school, had continued in college, and had maintained his use over the years since. Sam reported that currently he smokes two joints several eve-nings during the week (usually after using cocaine with friends earlier in the evening) and three to four joints on either Friday or Saturday evening (but not both). He stated that marijuana relaxed him and took the edge off after a long day at work. He also indicated that marijuana helped him to fall asleep at night and that not smoking contributed to a restless night and irritable feelings the following day. When asked to indicate differ-ences in himself on days he did not smoke versus days he did smoke, he replied that on smoking days he was more comfortable with himself and his world.

As implied above, Sam's current marijuana use was related in part to his cocaine use. Sam had first used crack cocaine in college, around a dozen times per year during his sophomore and junior years. He experi-enced a "scary high" when he used the cocaine ("scary" in the sense that he did not feel in control), but he asserted that this distress was more than offset by a euphoric feeling. He stopped using cocaine after his junior year because he had begun dating Joan, his wife-to-be, who did not use cocaine and was not comfortable with his using it.

Sam and Joan married 4 years ago, several years after they had met. They married one year after Sam's graduation with a degree in business accounting and immediately following Joan's graduation with a degree in nursing. They moved to a medium-sized city near their college town, where Sam accepted a position with an insurance company and Joan began working the evening shift at a public hospital. They were feeling good about their new jobs, but, according to Sam, they responded to their success differently. Joan devoted a considerable amount of energy to advancing her career and took courses toward a master's degree in nursing. Sam, on the other hand, felt he had delayed gratification long enough, and he wanted to live more in the here-and-now. He began meeting with coworkers after work (while Joan was working her evening shift) to use crack cocaine. His use, and corresponding expenditures, increased gradually. Now, a year later, he was spending more time away from home, was getting less sleep, and was feeling occasional nervousness. He admitted to occasional use of speedball, a mixture of cocaine and heroin, to reduce jittery nerves associated with coming down from cocaine highs. He also reported experiencing more and more anxiety and nervousness when using the cocaine. Joan over this period became progressively more conscious of Sam's erratic behavior, his missed time from work, and his increased spending habits. They both became aware that their marital relationship had deteriorated, although not to the point where either had voiced a desire for a separation or divorce. Their relationship had become characterized by a sense of detachment rather than closeness.

In summarizing his impressions of his current situation, Sam reiterated that he did not believe his drug use was a problem for him. Instead, he viewed it as his wife's problem, an outgrowth of her rigidity and overcontrolling style. He had agreed to come to the clinic simply to appease Joan and to get her to "lighten up." He cited evidence indicating he was not a drug abuser: no arrests, no problems at work (although he had been passed up for promotion on two occasions during the past 18 months), and no apparent health problems. He discounted as inconsequential his poor work attendance, spending time away from home using cocaine with his coworkers, difficulties maintaining cash flow, and a pervasive tired-out feeling. He left the session saying that he had met his obligation to his wife by coming and that he saw no need to continue contacts with the clinic.

The background material presented by Sam and his behavior throughout the intake session provided a number of signs of a drug abuser in the precontemplation stage. First of all, he was defensive and resisted any suggestions that his drug use was causing problems for him. Indeed, he felt that the problem was not his drug use, but rather the conservative and narrow viewpoints of his wife. He was, however, feeling pressure from his wife to seek treatment, and that was really the only reason he had attended the intake session. He was not invested in pursuing counseling, or even further evaluation.

THE CONTEMPLATION STAGE

An individual in the contemplation stage has begun thinking about changing his or her behavior but has not yet engaged in actual behavior change strategies. Among substance abusers, contemplators are seriously pondering quitting or reducing their substance use. Frequently their thoughts about change emanate from an awareness (internally or externally generated) of the disadvantages of continued alcohol or drug use. Such thoughts sometimes dovetail with positive thoughts about a drug-free lifestyle.

The contemplator has been described in more detail by Prochaska and DiClemente (1982). They characterized the contemplator as one who recognizes the existence of a problem, is working to understand or make sense of it, and is feeling distress and discomfort over this problem recognition. Prochaska and DiClemente (1982) view the contemplator as someone who is seeking to achieve a sense of mastery or control over the situation through a cognitive reappraisal.

An alcohol or drug abuser can remain in the contemplation stage for an indefinite period of time. The fact that a substance abuser enters treatment does not necessarily mean that he or she has left the stage of contemplation and has moved into the action stage. For many clients, entering treatment does not reflect action but rather a continuation of contemplation. When in treatment such clients are not necessarily resistant and can be open to discussing their concerns even if not ready to initiate action. These and some other common characteristics of the contemplator are summarized in Table 2.2.

The descriptions of contemplators in Table 2.2 have been borne out in clinical research. We return to DiClemente et al.'s (1991) large-scale study on the process of smoking cessation. Most of the individuals that DiClemente et al. (1991) studied were classified as being in the contemplation stage. These individuals were smokers who reported that they

TABLE 2.2. Common Characteristics of Individuals in the Contemplation Stage

Seeking to evaluate and understand their behavior

Distressed

Desirous of exerting control or mastery

Thinking about making change

Have not begun taking action and are not yet prepared to do so

Frequently have made attempts to change in the past

Evaluating pros and cons of their behavior and of making changes in it

Note. Adapted in part from Prochaska and DiClemente (1983, 1984); DiClemente and Hughes (1990); DiClemente et al. (1991); and Prochaska and DiClemente (1992).

were considering quitting during the following 6 months. They had not quit for more than a day during the past year and did not foresee quitting during the upcoming 30 days. Relative to the precontemplators, the contemplators had a history of more attempts to quit smoking, reported more concerns about wanting to quit, said they had fewer smoking temptations, had more confidence in their ability to quit, and identified fewer advantages and more disadvantages to smoking. The contemplators also described having previously resorted to more activities associated with quitting smoking. At a 1-month and 6-month follow-up, DiClemente et al. (1991) found that the contemplators, relative to the precontemplators, had initiated more quit attempts overall and that the percentage of contemplators who made a quit attempt in the past 30 days was greater than that for the sample of precontemplators.

DiClemente and Hughes (1990) identified a sample of contemplators in their study on alcohol abusers entering treatment. Those in the contemplative stage scored highest on the contemplation items from the Stages of Change Scale and lowest on precontemplation and action. A similar profile was found for a subgroup of the polysubstance abusers in the Carney and Kivlahan (1995) study. Thus, in both studies the contemplators were clients who were thinking about behavior change, but despite the fact that they were seeking treatment they scored below average on the action scale.

Contemplators in general are devoting serious thought to making changes in behavior but have not made a decision to take action. Contemplation is not only an interim stage preceding movement into preparation and action. While many shift from contemplation to preparation and action, there are those who remain in contemplation for extended periods of time and others who move back into precontemplation. One of the challenges facing the clinician is helping the contemplative client to move toward preparation and action.

Case Example of a Client in the Contemplation Stage

Maureen J is a 46-year-old divorced woman presenting at a community mental health center with concerns about her use of alcohol. She reports that she began drinking at around age 17, and says that she is drinking more than she would like and is thinking about quitting.

Regarding her background, Maureen is the oldest of three daughters. Her father was alcohol-dependent, and one of her sisters is a recovering alcoholic. There is no family history of psychiatric or drug problems. Maureen reports that she used some marijuana, LSD, and cocaine when she was in her twenties but not since. She married her high school sweetheart shortly after they had graduated. They divorced when she was 32, and they had no children. For the past 12 years Maureen has been working in a factory that produces windshield wipers. She has no history of psychiatric problems and has no previous treatment for alcohol abuse.

Maureen's drinking shows little variation from week to week. Almost all of her drinking occurs in a local tavern that is close to where she works and lives. Maureen is friendly with a number of other patrons there, some of whom are from work and some from other settings. On Mondays she generally is abstinent. On Tuesdays, Wednesdays, and Thursdays she typically consumes three to five bottles of beer each day. On weekends she drinks more heavily, about 10 to 12 beers daily. She acknowledges that in her drinking career she has experienced drinking binges while on vacations, has made rules to curtail drinking, tried to quit several times in the past, has missed work because of hangovers, and has experienced withdrawal from alcohol, predominantly in the form of mild shakes. Maureen saw these as fairly normal, stating that her drinking really is not much different from that of her friends. However, she is worried about several consequences of her drinking, specifically several recent blackouts, concerns expressed by her mother about her drinking, and feedback from her employer that she seemed to be missing more time from work recently and was not as sharp and on top of things during the morning as she had been in the past. In addition, although she has never been arrested for an alcohol-related offense, she drives home while under the influence of alcohol several times a week. These recent events, taken together, have put her in a position of thinking more about her alcohol use and the possibility of quitting. This is countered, in her mind, by the fact that she really has not been "burned" by her drinking and by her belief that important relationships with her friends will be negatively affected if she is not drinking and thus is not one of the gang. As such, she is unclear as to what she needs to do and about what she wants to do about her drinking. For that reason, she contacted the clinic to discuss these questions with a counselor.

Maureen's presentation reflects several characteristics commonly seen among persons contemplating a change in their drinking behavior. First and foremost, she is thinking about making a change, although she is ambivalent about the need to change and is concerned about how abstinence would influence her relationships with her friends. She is experiencing some distress (e.g., family concerns, employer comments on her missed time from work, driving under the influence of alcohol), although the fact that she has not experienced any major (from her point of view) negative consequences of drinking has lessened the impact of these events. In essence, she is in the midst of contemplating the pros and cons of her behavior and of making changes in her decisional balance that will determine whether she moves forward toward action or remains in contemplation or moves back to precontemplation.

THE PREPARATION STAGE

Individuals in the preparation stage are planning to initiate change in the near future and in many cases have learned valuable lessons from their past attempts at change and from failures associated with those efforts (Prochaska & DiClemente, 1992). The client in this stage has resolved the decision-making challenges faced during contemplation and has committed to a change plan soon to be implemented. Some common characteristics of persons in the preparation stage are shown in Table 2.3.

The inclusion of the preparation stage in the stages of change model has had an interesting history. Such a stage, called decision making, was originally proposed between contemplation and action. However, the analytic procedures used early on to evaluate data collected on the stages of change model suggested a four-step model (precontemplation, contem-

TABLE 2.3. Common Characteristics of Individuals in the Preparation Stage

Intending to change their behavior

Ready to change in terms of both attitude and behavior

On the verge of taking action

Engaged in the change process

Prepared to make firm commitments to follow through on the action option they choose

Making or having made the decision to change

Note. Adapted in part from DiClemente and Prochaska (1998); DiClemente et al. (1991); Prochaska and DiClemente (1992); and Prochaska, DiClemente, and Norcross (1992).

plation, action, and maintenance) (McConnaughy, Prochaska, & Velicer, 1983; McConnaughy, DiClemente, Prochaska, & Velicer, 1989). Later analyses, using an alternative data analytic approach felt to be more applicable, provided stronger support for the importance of and necessity for the preparation stage (DiClemente et al., 1991; Prochaska, DiClemente, & Norcross, 1992). Consequently, the present structure of the basic model includes five stages: precontemplation, contemplation, preparation, action, and maintenance.

Insights on clients in the preparation stage are provided in the study described by DiClemente et al. (1991), the investigation of processes of smoking cessation introduced earlier. The participants in that study who were classified as being in the preparation stage met two criteria: planning to quit within the next 30 days and had made a 24-hour quit attempt in the past year. Relative to precontemplators and contemplators, those in the preparation stage had a history of more prior attempts at quitting and had more quit attempts in the past year. In addition, those in preparation had higher levels of confidence in their ability to stop or maintain nonsmoking and of efficacy to abstain from smoking, relative to the precontemplators and contemplators. Evaluations of the pros and cons of smoking also differed as a function of the stage of change. In this regard, those in preparation rated the positives of smoking lower than those in precontemplation or contemplation. They also rated the negatives of smoking higher than did those in the precontemplation or contemplation stages.

When reevaluated 1 and 6 months later, individuals initially classified in the preparation stage were found to be engaged in a variety of activities associated with quitting smoking, and doing so to a greater degree than those previously classified as either precontemplators or contemplators. For example, those in preparation at baseline had initiated more quit attempts overall during follow-up and had greater percentages of individuals having made quit attempts and currently not smoking.

Consistent with the above behavioral indicators was the finding by DiClemente et al. (1991) that the individuals in preparation were engaging in a greater variety of experiential and behavioral change processes, relative to those in precontemplation or contemplation. In terms of experiential processes, those in preparation scored higher on the processes of consciousness raising (for example, seeking information about the addictive behavior, increasing awareness about one's problem behavior), environmental reevaluation (assessing the impact of the behavior on one's surroundings), and self-reevaluation (a personal reappraisal, in both affective and cognitive terms, of the problem and its impact on the person). In the domain of behavioral processes, those in preparation scored higher on self-liberation (choosing and committing to change), counterconditioning (making changes in the conditioned stimuli that influence behavior), reinforcement management (altering the contingencies that influence behavior), stimulus control (restructuring the environment to reduce the likelihood of a particular conditioned stimulus occurring), and dramatic relief. Taken together, individuals in preparation are high on dimensions related to both contemplation and action. This pattern was reflected in the DiClemente and Hughes (1990) presentation of a "participation" profile among alcoholics. Clients in this group were low on precontemplation and highest on contemplation and action. A nearly identical pattern was found by Carney and Kivlahan (1995) among polysubstance abusers.

Case Example of a Client in the Preparation Stage

Tim L is a 34-year-old single man who attended an intake session at an outpatient drug treatment program. He was self-referred and had called to set up the appointment several days earlier. As part of a telephone prescreen, Tim indicated that he had been abusing amphetamines for years.

Tim presented at the intake session appearing tired and drained. Nevertheless, he was responsive and fully engaged throughout the session.

He began immediately with a description of his current drug use. Specifically, Tim outlined a daily pattern of amphetamine use designed to aid him in dealing with a variety of daily tasks and activities. He reported that two years earlier he decided to enroll at a local junior college. At the time, he had been working an evening shift (4:30 P.M.–1:00 A.M.) at an office supply warehouse, loading trucks that would depart the following morning to make deliveries to local businesses throughout the city. In addition, Tim was working several hours a day (up to 6 or 8 on days he did not have classes) as a car mechanic at a friend's garage, being paid "off the books." During school sessions, he sought to enroll in classes scheduled for the morning hours.

Tim reported that his use of the amphetamines, purchased regularly from a "safe contact who didn't work the streets," was an effort to "keep him going" and "on top of things." He reported that he generally felt this strategy was working, but that increasingly he was feeling "on edge," "irritable," and "just plain zapped." Although not described in his telephone prescreen, Tim at the intake also described daily use of marijuana, generally one or two joints when he got home at night. Further, he reported that throughout the day he was "almost always" drinking coffee and, when permissible, smoking cigarettes.

Tim's decision to contact the clinic was a difficult one because, he reported, it suggested he wasn't in charge of the situation. He was fearful that "everything would come crumbling down" and that his hopes of using his coursework to obtain a business or managerial position would not be realized. Tim suspected that his work at the supply warehouse was viewed as average at best, citing some tardiness and also periodic errors on getting orders onto the correct delivery trucks. However, he did not feel his employment was in jeopardy. At school he felt he was not performing up to his potential. He noted his social life was not affected because he didn't have one.

The decision by Tim to seek help coincided with several other decisions. First, he had decided to work at the garage only on days when he did not have classes. Second, he determined that his use of amphetamines needed to be terminated. He previously felt that he could simply reduce such use and tailor it to particular situations. He had made several efforts at reduction in the past, with no real effect. Third, while clear on the need to stop his use of marijuana and cigarettes as well, he wondered about the timing. Tim was concerned that stopping use of all three at once might make more difficult the termination of his main drug of concern. Finally, Tim reported that he had set the initiation of treatment as the starting point for making change, however recommended and scheduled by his counselor.

Several aspects of Tim's presentation stood out. He was clearly ready to change, certainly in terms of attitude and seemingly on the verge in terms of behavior. He had begun to take action by virtue of initiating his clinic appointment. While not yet modifying his substance use, he was evidencing a firm commitment to the change process. To all outward appearance, he had engaged himself in the process of change and was prepared to proceed accordingly.

THE ACTION STAGE

As described by Prochaska, DiClemente, and Norcross (1992), "action is the stage in which individuals modify their behavior, experiences, or environment in order to overcome their problems" (p. 1104). In this regard, there are two central features that characterize persons in the action stage. The first is a firm and clear decision or commitment to change. The second is the appearance of active behavioral manifestations of the commitment to change. Most typically these change attempts are reflected in individuals' efforts to make modifications in their behavioral patterns or in their environments. A listing of some characteristics common among people in the action stage is provided in Table 2.4.

Several studies have been conducted in an effort to empirically iden-

---

TABLE 2.4. Common Characteristics of Individuals in the Action Stage

Client has decided to make change.

Client has verbalized or otherwise demonstrated a firm commitment to making change.

Efforts to modify behavior and/or one's environment are being taken.

Client presents motivation and effort to achieve behavioral change.

Client has committed to making change and is involved in the change process.

Client is willing to follow suggested strategies and activities to change.

Note. Adapted in part from Prochaska and DiClemente (1984, 1992) and DiClemente and Hughes (1990).

tify characteristics of people in the action stage. An early study by Prochaska and DiClemente (1983) involved the evaluation of over 850 persons who responded to newspaper articles and advertisements for a study on making changes in smoking behavior. Recent smoking quitters, representing persons in the action stage, were defined as those who had quit smoking within 6 months of participating in the study. All subjects were evaluated according to the extent to which they were using different processes or mechanisms related to change. These processes, discussed in detail by Prochaska and DiClemente (1984), include consciousness raising, self-liberation, stimulus control, and helping relationships (relationships, including the therapeutic relationship, that provide support and inputs to making change), and persons in different stages of change would be expected to score differentially on these change processes. As an example, precontemplators would be expected to score low on most of the change processes, since they are not thinking about change. Contemplators, on the other hand, might be expected to score particularly high on consciousness raising.

In studying the individuals classified as being in the action phase, Prochaska and DiClemente (1983) found that these subjects scored highest on the processes of change labeled self-liberation, counterconditioning, stimulus control, reinforcement management, and helping relationships, relative to subjects classified as precontemplators or contemplators. Similar findings have been reported by Ahijevych and Wewers (1992). Prochaska, Velicer, DiClemente, and Fava (1988) showed that these five processes reflect a more general cluster of processes that includes activities with the aim of behavior change and of using others as resources for support and encouragement in the behavior change efforts.

Monitoring the extent of use of the varied processes of change across the stages of change model can provide information on when and where a particular process will be predominant. In conducting research on this topic, Prochaska, Velicer, Guadagnoli, Rossi, and DiClemente (1991) noted that reinforcement management is the first process that predominates for clients in the action stage. Prochaska et al. (1991) also found that the processes of self-reevaluation and stimulus control peak in the middle phase of the action stage, providing further support for viewing these processes as particularly relevant to this stage.

DiClemente and Hughes (1990) and Carney and Kivlahan (1995) identified an action stage profile in samples of alcohol and other substance abusers. Their clinical assessments in each case included administration of the URICA (described in Chapter 3) to determine scores on precontemplation, contemplation, action, and maintenance scales. One of the profiles that emerged from DiClemente and Hughes's analyses of the URICA scale scores reflected persons high on the action stage score. DiClemente and Hughes called this profile the participation cluster. Because these clients scored well above average on both the action and contemplation scales, it seems they are invested in behavior change and are actively engaged in that effort. The clients also scored above average on the maintenance scale. As would be expected, their scores on the precontemplation scale were low.

A subgroup of the polydrug users in the Carney and Kivlahan (1995) sample also exhibited a distinct pattern of scores that was similar to the participation cluster described by DiClemente and Hughes (1990): URICA scores were highest on the contemplation and action scales, above average on the maintenance scale, and well below average on the precontemplation scale. These polydrug users, then, can be described as clients who are not only thinking seriously about change but who also are actively engaged in the change process.

Taken together, these findings suggest that individuals in the action stage have decided to make changes in their behavior, have committed to making these changes, and have begun taking action to effect the changes they want to achieve. Action-stage clients are motivated and ready to initiate steps to produce change, and the changes that occur in the action stage typically are the most dramatic and overt of those that occur in any of the four stages. The action phase most commonly has a duration of 3 to 6 months.

Case Example of a Client in the Action Stage

Paul J is a 34-year-old single man who attended an intake evaluation session at an addictions treatment center. He reported that he had been using multiple substances in various combinations since junior high school (currently he was using alcohol, cocaine, and marijuana). Further, he had decided that he wanted to be abstinent from all substance use, including alcohol, and immediately wanted to start taking the steps necessary to achieve this goal.

Paul's demeanor during his evaluation was serious, compliant, accommodating, and eager. He reported that he had used a variety of drugs since his junior high school years. The listing he provided included alcohol, marijuana, cocaine, LSD, peyote, stimulants, inhalants, and depressants. Paul noted that during different periods of his life he had been using different combinations of these drugs. For example, during junior high school he was using mainly alcohol and marijuana. During high school he began using cocaine regularly (around once a week). Immediately after high school he began spending much of his time with friends who were using inhalants and depressants. During his twenties his drug use predominantly revolved around the hallucinogens (e.g., LSD, peyote) and stimulants. Finally, Paul described that during the past 6 years his drug use had been restricted for the most part to almost daily use of marijuana and alcohol, and use of cocaine approximately four times a week. He noted that he occasionally would also use stimulants other than cocaine, but that such use was infrequent (maybe once a month, he estimated).

Paul's family, especially a brother and a sister, were concerned that his drug use was causing him to be "stuck" in his relationships and employment. Paul acknowledged that his drug use over the past decade had precluded the development of significant or long-term relationships with women (and often with friends more generally) and that he had difficulties maintaining a job. In fact, according to Paul, he had spent most of the past 10 years either underemployed, on unemployment benefits, or on welfare support. The status that bothered him most was underemployment because he felt he was capable of more challenging positions that would provide stimulation as well as better salaries. He noted, with some pride, that his drug use had not led to problems in his physical health (at least, as far as he was aware), accidents, or arrests. It was the absence of problems in these areas that he had used in the past as evidence that he did not have a problem with drug use.

Paul's current alcohol and drug use occurred with various combinations of acquaintances from a core group of around 15 persons. Sometimes he would get together with two or three of these individuals and they would (generally) go to someone's apartment to drink or use drugs. He would meet these people at one or two local spots where members of the group tended to congregate. Paul did not spend much time with these individuals beyond these specific drug use contexts. He would visit the local congregating settings in the mid- to late afternoon when not working, and after work when he was employed.

Paul at his intake session could not identify the precipitating circumstances that led to his decision to quit his alcohol and drug use. He did note that on numerous occasions in the past he had made the decision to terminate use of one or more—but not all—of the substances he was using at the time. For example, on a handful of occasions he had decided to stop using cocaine but did not feel at those times the need to make changes in his use of marijuana or alcohol. These past decisions regarding behavior change were short-lived, and Paul said that he did not believe his heart was in making long-term changes at that time. More often, he reported, he was responding to some acute illness associated with recent drug use or greater than usual complaints from his family.

This time, however, he said it was different. As he put it, now he "really" had decided to change and indeed had already implemented several steps in this regard. As an indication of this heightened commitment, Paul had not used any alcohol or drugs during the preceding 5 days and he had attended his intake session. Paul had also begun to attend meetings of Alcoholics Anonymous, and in other contexts had begun to seek out and spend time with acquaintances not using drugs. Also unique to his current decision was the commitment to stop *all* drug use. Paul felt now that it was necessary for him to be abstinent from alcohol as well as all other substances.

Some of the more common characteristics of clients in the action stage were evident in Paul's intake presentation. First and foremost, he was verbalizing a firm decision to initiate and achieve behavioral changes in his use of alcohol and other drugs. Second, he was ready to collaborate with his counselor to initiate steps to become sober. In fact, Paul had already initiated some steps on his own before his session and had been abstinent for several days. By all appearances he was motivated and committed to make changes.

THE MAINTENANCE STAGE

The stage of maintenance is characterized predominantly by two endeavors. The first is sustaining and further incorporating changes achieved during the action stage, and the second is avoiding relapse. Persons in the maintenance stage have accomplished at least some minimal amount of change as a function of successful efforts exerted during the action stage. A listing of some characteristics often reported by individuals in maintenance is given in Table 2.5.

Since sustaining change often entails continued use of techniques for initiating change, it is not surprising that the processes of change used

TABLE 2.5. Common Characteristics of Individuals in the Maintenance Stage

Client is working to sustain changes achieved to date.

Considerable attention is focused on avoiding slips or relapses.

Client may describe fear or anxiety regarding relapse and facing a high risk for relapse situation.

Less frequent but often intense temptations to use substances or return to substance use may be faced.

Note. Adapted in part from Prochaska and DiClemente (1984, 1992) and DiClemente and Hughes (1990).

most by persons in maintenance overlap with processes frequently observed in the action stage. Most noteworthy among persons in maintenance are the processes of counterconditioning, stimulus control, self-liberation, and self-management (Ahijevych & Wewers, 1992; DiClemente & Prochaska, 1982; Prochaska & DiClemente, 1983, 1986). The overlap between the action and maintenance stages on predominant processes highlights that maintenance is not static but instead an active and vital endeavor.

Given the overlap in primary change processes, one might wonder about how to tell if a person is in action versus maintenance. For research purposes, investigators have operationalized the onset of maintenance as 6 months following some successful action, such as the last drug use or drink (e.g., Prochaska, DiClemente, & Norcross, 1992). Clinically speaking, action might be viewed as a period during which efforts are taken to effect change and get such change established, with maintenance occurring after initial change-related efforts have stabilized. The selection of this 6-month point was also guided by indications in the relapse literature that the vast majority of relapses occur during this time frame.

Since addictive behaviors are complex, multifaceted problems, therapists and clients often work to break a problem domain down into more manageable components. For example, consider the case of a polydrug abuser who mainly uses cocaine, marijuana, and alcohol. He or she may further report that cocaine use is creating the majority of problems in his or her life but that eventually he or she wants to terminate all substance use. It may be that the therapist and client agree to focus on the cocaine use first and utilize successes in that arena to subsequently terminate the use of marijuana and alcohol. In such a scenario, the client might achieve abstinence from cocaine using a set of change strategies and utilize them successfully for an extended period of time such that they become part of a maintenance stage. Meanwhile, the client might start action-related strategies for cessation of marijuana and alcohol use. In this manner, he or she may be in a stage of maintenance regarding cocaine use but in an action state regarding marijuana and alcohol use.

While there may not be an unequivocal definition for when one departs from action and embarks on maintenance, there is more certainty on what represents a failure in either action or maintenance, and that is relapse. When a person relapses and uses again a particular substance, it is clear that there was a breakdown in the strategies that had been employed previously to sustain abstinence. At such a point, and as discussed in Chapter 1, such persons might attempt to "recycle" themselves by reinitiating contemplation, preparation, or action. Alternatively, some individuals might be sufficiently discouraged that they revert back to a stage of precontemplation.

A final issue surrounding the stage of maintenance is the question of whether a person ever successfully leaves this stage. In the abstract, the answer is yes, when the individual's temptations to use are at a level of zero and when the person's confidence about not using drugs is 100% (Prochaska & DiClemente, 1986). More practically, however, it probably makes some sense to view these individuals as continuing to maintain and thus remaining aware of risks or challenges to their maintenance of a particular change in behavior.

Case Example of a Client in the Maintenance Stage

Angela M is a 47-year-old woman who quit drinking around 11 months ago. Prior to then she had been drinking heavily and problematically for over 20 years, experiencing over that period a variety of negative alcohol-related consequences.

Angela began drinking in high school, and her drinking at that time was limited to weekend drinking with friends. However, even then she reported she was drinking too much and over time began to experience hangovers and some difficulties remembering events from the preceding evening while drinking. Following high school she attended a local community college and continued drinking in this pattern, with the exception that she might also drink on some weekday evening as well. Despite taking many risks, she reports, she managed to avoid any alcohol-related arrests during this time, such as driving under the influence. Angela does note, though, that she probably would have done better in school and performed better on her part-time jobs had she not been drinking so much.

Throughout high school and while attending community college, Angela lived at home with her parents and one younger brother. While her parents were upset with the frequency of her drinking, she never had the sense they were particularly concerned about it. After completing her coursework, Angela took a position as an engineering technician, which entailed serving as an assistant to company staff working on building renovation plans. Since the job was not within commuting distance from her home, she moved into an apartment with a girlfriend she had known in college.

Angela reports that in the following years there were several changes in her drinking. For example, she found that she could consume relatively large amounts of alcohol, considerably more than her friends and acquaintances. She also found that she was consuming a larger array of alcoholic beverages, including strong mixed drinks. Finally, Angela reported that she was not convinced she had much "direction" in life and worried that she might not find a partner to settle down with.

Angela characterizes the next 20 years as a "blur," despite several notable life events. For example, she initiated four job changes, two of which were promotions professionally. The other two were for "changes in scenery." In addition, she met a man, Peter, whom she lived with for several years and then married when she was 37. Angela describes this relationship then and currently as the most valued aspect of her life.

The reason those 20 years were described as a blur is that her drinking continued to the point where she was drinking around 6 ounces of alcohol most evenings, and more on weekends. Peter also drank frequently, but rarely as heavily, and he only occasionally confronted her about her drinking. Gradually, though, Angela reported an awareness of more and more signals that she needed to cut back, the most pronounced being a pair of arrests for driving under the influence of alcohol at ages 40 and 42. After the first arrest, she reports she cut back considerably but gradually returned to her prearrest level of drinking. The second arrest was followed in time with three attempts at outpatient alcoholism treatment, at ages 42, 43, and 44. The first two treatment endeavors were "helpful" and led to a fair amount of abstinence and many fewer heavy drinking days. However, the changes never lasted as long as she wanted— perhaps, she reports, because she was not fully committed to abstaining completely. Her third treatment, at age 44, "took hold" in that she found her resolve stronger than ever and her working relationship with her counselor particularly helpful and positive. They focused extensively on a number of approaches to achieving stable abstinence, including a detailed functional analysis of her drinking (the determinants, immediate and longer-term consequences, expected negative effects and benefits of drinking, and so on), development of alternatives to drinking (including stress management, avoiding situations associated with previous heavy drinking, coping with cravings and urges, and drink refusal skills), the inclusion of Peter in portions of treatment to incorporate his support and encouragement, and the development of plans to prevent relapse or at least to minimize drinking, should a slip occur.

Angela's treatment entailed mostly weekly individual and group sessions for almost 10 months, followed by mostly individual sessions on a less frequent basis. While she experienced some setbacks, she generally rebounded quickly, and, perhaps more importantly, she felt she learned valuable "sobriety lessons" from such events. Eventually, she and her counselor determined that they comfortably could move to scheduling monthly appointments. They further agreed that Angela could call and touch base prior to the scheduled appointment time, and if all was going well they could cancel the appointment and reschedule for a month later.

It was at this point that Angela was phasing herself more fully into the maintenance stage. During recent years she had taken considerable action to cease her drinking, especially during her third outpatient treatment. Angela had incorporated a variety of change strategies that she had been using successfully, following an early period of trial-and-error in the application of these strategies. Now her attention was focused on what she called "cruise control," whereby she could step back from the vigilance associated with skill acquisition and application and instead let much of that behavior occur more naturally. She emphasized that "cruise control" still entailed paying close attention to her environment, including attention to her own thoughts and feelings. Further, Angela still spent time anticipating drinking situations and reviewing in advance her plans to deal with such situations. Even with close to a year of abstinence, she experienced periodic thoughts and temptations regarding alcohol use, although she was pleased that she could not really classify them as cravings. Finally, it was Angela's sense that she would always need to be in a state of full awareness regarding potential challenges to her abstinence and that she would never be in a position to take her sobriety for granted.

CLINICAL ISSUES RELEVANT TO THE PRECONTEMPLATION, CONTEMPLATION, AND PREPARATION STAGES

As we noted earlier, persons in the precontemplation and contemplation stages are not taking action toward changing their substance use. Individuals in preparation have made the decision and are already planning on making changes in their behavior, although some resistance may remain. The lack of decisional action unfortunately has been thought to reflect "denial" and/or "resistance," and traditionally it has been argued that a primary task of the clinician is to confront denial or resistance in order to break through it. Successful confrontation is presumed to set the stage for the individual to take action regarding his or her substance use disorder.

In this section we discuss denial and resistance in greater depth. We first define the terms and then describe how they are assumed to be manifested in the treatment process. Next, alternative ways of conceptualizing denial and resistance are discussed. We emphasize motivational interviewing, which involves the use of a variety of clinical techniques to help individuals mobilize their own motivations and resources to overcome their ambivalence and begin to create behavioral change (Miller & Rollnick, 1991).

Denial

Although Paolino and McCrady (1977), among others, have called denial the most misused term in the substance abuse literature, denial nevertheless is a cornerstone of many models of rehabilitation for persons with substance use disorders. Chafetz (1970) identified denial as one of the alcoholic's most characteristic defense mechanisms. He wrote that "denial constitutes the main method by which alcoholics deal with life" (Chafetz, 1970, p. 10), and similar impressions have been offered regarding persons who abuse drugs other than alcohol (e.g., Washton, 1987). Further, clinicians say denial is among the most difficult problems they face in working with clients (Metzger, 1988). In fact, one proposed definition of alcoholism, published in the *Journal of the American Medical Association* (Morse & Flavin, 1992), included a component called "distortions in thinking, most notably denial" (p. 1012). The committee developing the definition used denial in their formulation "not only in the psychoanalytic sense of a single psychologic defense mechanism disavowing the significance of events but more broadly to include a range of psychologic maneuvers that decrease awareness of the fact that alcohol use is the cause of a person's problems rather than a solution to those problems. Denial becomes an integral part of the disease and is nearly always a major obstacle to recovery" (p. 1013).

Denial is rooted in the psychoanalytic literature on defense mechanisms, which are viewed as unconscious processes used by an individual to alleviate emotional conflict and anxiety. Vaillant (1977) organized the variety of defense mechanisms (e.g., distortion, projection, repression, suppression) according to the level of maturity they reflect and their importance to the degree of psychopathology. Denial was placed in the category of least mature defense mechanisms. As described by Vaillant (1977), denial's primary component is a distorted perception of reality. As such, denial entails negating or refusing thoughts, external feedback, and other forms of awareness about a behavior that, if fully conscious and "rational," would be intolerable to the individual.

Anderson (1981) provided one of the more comprehensive discussions of denial. He used the term denial to designate "a wide repertoire of psychological defenses and maneuvers that alcoholic persons unwittingly set up to protect themselves from the realization that they do in fact have a drinking problem" (p. 11), or by extension, a problem with any psychoactive substance. As with defense mechanisms more generally, denial was seen as an unconscious (unwitting) process. Moreover, denial can also operate within the substance abuser's family or other support systems.

Anderson (1981) identified a variety of the defensive maneuvers that are most typically observed, including simple denial, minimizing, blaming, rationalizing, intellectualizing, diversion, and hostility. These seven forms of denial are outlined in Table 2.6. In discussing these manifestations of denial, Anderson provided two of its other features. The first is that denial is automatic and not simply lying or willfully deceptive. Instead the denial is an outgrowth of a firmly entrenched state of self-delusion. The second feature of denial, according to Anderson, is that it is progressive. He observes that "by the time an individual's illness is sufficiently advanced that the problem appears serious to others, an elaborate system of defenses has usually been built up" (p. 13). Thus, as the severity of alcoholism increases, the complexity and intractability of the denial increases comparably.

TABLE 2.6. Common Forms of Denial

Simple denial—insists that alcohol or drug use is not a problem despite clear evidence to the contrary.

Minimizing—acknowledges some level of a substance abuse problem but discounts it as not significant or serious.

Blaming—projects responsibility for the problem externally, on other people or events and circumstances. Personal responsibility is abdicated.

Rationalizing—uses "alibis, excuses, justifications and other explanations" (Anderson, 1981, p. 12) to account for the substance abuse.

Intellectualizing—addresses the substance abuse in an intellectual, analytic, and unemotional manner.

Diversion—avoids the substance abuse issue by distracting attention from the topic.

Hostility—responds to others who raise the issue of substance abuse with anger, irritation, and/or scorn (as examples), with the intent of dissuading others from raising the topic.

Note. Data from Anderson (1981, pp. 11–12).

Resistance

Another term frequently encountered in the treatment literature on substance abuse is resistance. A hallmark construct in the psychoanalytic literature for decades, resistance was defined by Fenichel (1945) as "everything that prevents the patient from producing material derived from the unconscious" (p. 27). The concept of resistance is "understood in psychoanalysis as the process through which any action, emotion, or thought comes to interfere with the patient's becoming conscious . . . of previously unconscious mental processes and contents" (Lotti, 1987, p. 88).

More recently, therapists use the term "resistance" more generally to refer to client behaviors that they view as antitherapeutic (Turkat & Meyer, 1982). As such, resistance is seen as occurring on both conscious and unconscious levels. While resistance may have the goal of avoiding uncomfortable feelings such as anxiety or guilt, resistance also can refer to the client who is unmotivated for change. Representative of this view are Lazarus and Fay (1982), who state that "resistant patients are neither people who 'do not want help' nor are 'deliberate saboteurs,' but instead people for whom exploration and change are difficult, painful, and even dangerous" (p. 200).

In an effort to specify better the construct of resistance, several investigators have identified subcategories of resistance and have applied the term to particular diagnostic domains or therapeutic approaches. Sandler, Holder, and Dare (1970), for example, identified 10 forms of resistance that may occur during psychotherapy (e.g., transference resistance, resistance due to secondary gain, resistance related to specific behavior change techniques). In addition, Cavaiola (1984) proposed a set of stages of resistance that characterizes drunk driving recidivists, and Weissberg and Levay (1981) applied Sandler et al.'s (1970) forms of resistance to conjoint sex therapy. Examinations of resistance in the context of particular therapeutic approaches have been provided for family therapy (Anderson & Stewart, 1983; Larson & Talley, 1977; Will, 1983), marital therapy (Gurman, 1984; Spinks & Birchler, 1982), and group therapy (Balgopal & Hull, 1973; Muhleman, 1987). Similarly, in addition to discussions of resistance in psychoanalytic psychotherapy (Chessick, 1974; Greenson, 1967), the construct has been described in relation to behavior therapy (Jahn & Lichstein, 1980), cognitive-behavior therapy (Golden, 1983), and rational-emotive therapy (Ellis, 1983a, 1983b, 1984, 1985).

Reconceptualizing Denial and Resistance

As noted above, denial and resistance are concepts frequently used to explain why clients do not succeed in treatment. As such, it is the client traits of resistance and denial that lead to a treatment failure. However, there are significant difficulties in empirically documenting the validity of a trait model in accounting for treatment responsivity (see Miller, 1985). Among the components of the trait model that have *not* been substantiated, according to Miller (1985), are that denial is more frequently seen among alcoholics than among other clinical populations and that denial is directly related to treatment outcome.

Miller (1985) and Miller and Rollnick (1991) have argued that the use of constructs such as denial and resistance has not advanced our knowledge about addictive behavior or its treatment. As an alternative, they have focused on motivation. Miller (1985) notes that the term "motivation" frequently is viewed as the flip side of denial and resistance. So, according to Miller (1985), an important endeavor in the treatment of addictive behaviors is to work toward maximizing the occurrence of behaviors related to resolution of the substance use problem. In this regard, a "motivational intervention" would refer to any "operation that increases the probability of entering, continuing, and complying with an active change strategy" (Miller, 1985, p. 88). Miller (1985) originally outlined a series of motivational interventions that potentially could be used to promote change, including giving advice, providing feedback, setting goals, role playing, continuing contacts, manipulating external contingencies, providing choices, and decreasing the attractiveness of problem behavior. More recently, Miller and Rollnick (1991) summarized these and other strategies as "building blocks" that can be applied as part of the clinician's effort to engender productive change in an individual's addictive behavior. These strategies, described in detail in Miller and Rollnick (1991), are listed in Table 2.7.

It is useful to describe several of these strategies in the context of the stages of change model, particularly the stages of precontemplation and contemplation. Precontemplators, as noted earlier, are characterized by lack of awareness of a drug problem and evidence that drug use is contributing to dysfunction. As a result, one objective of motivational interventions with clients in the precontemplation stage often is to make more salient the effects of their drug use on their lives. Among contemplators who are ambivalent about the level of the problem or making change, a major goal of motivational interventions is to emphasize the pros of reduced or zero use and the cons of continued use at existing levels and to encourage the taking of steps that will lead to action.

The intervention of decreasing attractiveness, as an example, would be applicable to working with clients in either the precontemplation or contemplation stages. Decreasing the attractiveness of the drug potentially makes it easier for precontemplators to become aware of and acknowledge the negatives of drug use. Similarly, contemplators may be able to tip the balance in favor of the disadvantages of drug use and consequently move toward action to change their drug use.

Providing choice is another intervention with potential therapeutic

TABLE 2.7. Motivational Strategies for Promoting Change among Persons with Addictive Behaviors

Giving advice	Practicing empathy
Removing barriers	Providing feedback
Providing choice	Clarifying goals
Decreasing desirability	Active helping

Note. From Miller and Rollnick (1991, p. 20). Copyright 1991 by The Guilford Press. Reprinted by permission.

relevance for precontemplators and contemplators. In the case of precontemplators, identifying options for the client may help diffuse the resentments that arise when an authority figure or significant other has applied pressure on the client to seek treatment. If the client believes he or she has a choice in directions that can be taken, then the accompanying sense that he or she can prescribe and guide the course of action may result in initiating critical steps toward change. Similarly, the contemplator wavering about change may use the availability of several options as a way of initiating steps toward action.

These and numerous other intervention strategies are discussed in greater detail throughout this volume. For now, they are introduced in the context of interventions relevant to the processes of changing behavior.

CLINICAL ISSUES RELEVANT TO THE ACTION AND MAINTENANCE STAGES

The clinical tasks associated with working with clients in the action and maintenance stages are appropriately different from those faced when clients are in the precontemplation, contemplation, and preparation stages. As noted earlier in this chapter, the client in the action stage has begun to take steps to change behavior, and the client in the maintenance stage has reached some initial success in achieving his or her behavior change goals and is seeking now to maintain those goals. Below we identify some of the issues that arise in working with clients in these two stages and preview some of the strategies that can be used in addressing these issues. These issues and strategies are discussed in much greater detail throughout the remainder of this volume.

Clients in the action stages generally have developed a plan for change and have begun to implement it. As highlighted by DiClemente (1991), they often use treatment to make a public commitment to action, to obtain some external confirmation of their plan, to seek support, to gain greater self-efficacy, and in many cases to create artificial external monitors of their behavior. Helping clients increase their sense of self-efficacy is a particularly important task of the action stage. Focusing on clients' successful activities, reaffirming their decisions, and helping them to make intrinsic attributions of success can affect their self-efficacy eval-

TABLE 2.8. Representative Clinical Strategies Applicable to Clients in the Action Stage

Maintain client engagement in treatment.

Support a realistic view of change through small, successive steps.

Acknowledge the difficulties encountered in the early stages of change.

Help client identify high-risk situations through a functional analysis and develop appropriate coping strategies to overcome these.

Assist client in finding new reinforcers of positive change.

Help client assess whether he or she has strong family and social support.

Note. From Miller (1999).

uations. A sampling of clinical strategies potentially applicable for use with clients in the action stage is shown in Table 2.8.

Clients in the maintenance stage are seeking to firmly establish their new behavioral patterns and avoid a return to substance use. Sustaining behavior change can be very difficult, and relapses often occur. A sample of strategies available for use with clients in the maintenance stage is shown in Table 2.9. These and other matters are discussed thoroughly in upcoming chapters on clinical interventions. The issue of relapse, and clinical responses to such events, is addressed in detail in Chapter 9.

SUMMARY

- Persons in the precontemplation stage generally are unaware or ignorant of their drug use problem. If aware, they are not thinking seriously about their drug use or about making changes in it.
- Researchers have identified a group of individuals labeled ambivalent. These are individuals who rate highest on precontemplation but also above average on contemplation, action, and maintenance stages of change.
- Contemplators have started to think about making changes in their behavior, but as yet have not made the decision to change or initiated actual behavior change strategies.
- Individuals in the preparation stage have resolved the decision-making issues faced in contemplation and are planning to initiate change in the near future.
- Clients in the action stage are characterized by a firm decision to

TABLE 2.9. Representative Clinical Strategies Applicable to Clients in the Maintenance Stage

Help client identify and sample drug-free sources of satisfaction (i.e., develop new reinforcers).

Support lifestyle changes.

Affirm client's resolve and self-efficacy.

Help client practice and apply new coping strategies to avoid a return to drug use.

Maintain supportive contact.

Note. From Miller (1999).

make change and by evidence of active, overt behavioral manifestations of the commitment to change.

• Several specific processes of change tend to be the most useful matches for clients in the action stage: self-liberation, counterconditioning, stimulus control, reinforcement management, and helping relationships.

• Research has identified a cluster of individuals who appear to be in the action stage. Based on the URICA, they score high on the contemplation and action stages of change and low on precontemplation.

• Clients in the maintenance stage are predominantly focused on sustaining changes and on avoiding relapse.

• Processes used considerably by persons in maintenance are counterconditioning, stimulus control, self-liberation, and self-management.

• The lack of action that characterizes precontemplators and contemplators traditionally has been called denial or resistance.

• Denial has been described as a core strategy used by substance abusers to deal with life and to avoid awareness of their substance use problem. Resistance has been operationalized as countertherapeutic behaviors directed toward minimizing uncomfortable feelings.

• Focusing on the construct of motivation may be an alternative to the focus on denial and resistance. A variety of motivational interventions, including offering advice, giving feedback, providing choices, and decreasing the attractiveness of problem behavior, have been identified by Miller and his colleagues.

• Motivation, in terms of acknowledging problems, making decisions to change, initiating change, and maintaining changes, is an important component of each of the stages of change.

3

ASSESSMENT

Assessment is a critical concern in all substance abuse treatment settings. Its importance is underlined by the attention directed to it in the Joint Commission on Accreditation of Healthcare Organization's (JCAHO; 1996) standards on health care. However, defining assessment, though it is so widely practiced, is difficult. In this book we use as a general definition of assessment the collection and use of information to obtain an understanding of an individual (or couple or family), usually for purposes of treatment planning, modification, and evaluation. Therefore, assessment may occur before, during, or following any defined period of treatment (e.g., Donovan, 1988; Sobell, Sobell, & Nirenberg, 1988; Sobell, Toneatto, & Sobell, 1994).

A review and copies of many of the most important assessment measures used in alcohol and drug treatment are readily available (Allen & Columbus, 1995). Rather than reviewing these measures, in this chapter we will show ways to identify systematically an individual's stage of change. No matter how interesting the idea of "stage of change," it can have practical value only if it can be measured. From there, we will identify and discuss a variety of measures that have particular relevance to the assessment of individuals in different stages of change. The ultimate goal of this presentation is to increase understanding of how such assessments can be used to improve treatment planning for individuals in different stages of change, which is discussed in Chapter 4.

MEASURING THE STAGE OF CHANGE

As we noted in Chapter 1, the stages of change model was developed to reflect an individual's attitudes, intentions, and behaviors that are associated with the process of changing a given problem behavior. According to this model, the change process is best represented by a series of discrete periods, or stages, that a person passes through. Key features of stage models are the assumptions that discrete segments of a process can be defined and that being in one segment precludes being in another at the same time.

Several instruments to measure stage of change (recently summarized and critiqued by Carey, Purnine, Maisto, & Carey, 1999) have been developed. All involve respondents reporting on their perceptions and attitudes toward change or on their behavior in the recent past relevant to the problem behavior. Intentions regarding engaging in the behavior in the near future also may be part of the measure.

One of the major ways to measure a person's stage of change is to classify the client into one of the stages of change, based on how the individual answers five simple questions. This measure is called the staging algorithm and is presented first. Thereafter we will discuss the University of Rhode Island Change Assessment Scale, the Stages of Change Readiness and Treatment Eagerness Scale, and the Readiness to Change Questionnaire. Each of these latter three measures provides a quantitative score for each stage of change, based on the individual's responses to questionnaire items. The resulting scores enable one to define a person as being in one "dominant" stage of change or to construct a readiness to change "profile" based on the individual's score for each of the stages.

Staging Algorithm

In the staging algorithm procedure, respondents are asked to answer five simple questions, and a combination of their responses is scored according to predetermined rules (Prochaska & DiClemente, 1992). These scores allow one to classify subjects as in precontemplation, contemplation, preparation, action, or maintenance. The questions concern (1) whether the subject still engages in the problem behavior (in this case, smoking), (2) whether he or she is considering quitting in the next 6 months, (3) whether he or she is planning to quit in the next 30 days, (4) whether he or she has stopped smoking for at least 24 hours in the past year, and, if he or she has quit, (5) for how long. Subjects can be classified in one and only one stage of change. The staging algorithm has been used in studies that have provided strong evidence for the ability of stage of change to predict treatment outcomes, which is essential to the argument that stage of change has clinical utility (Belding, Iguchi, & Lamb, 1997).

University of Rhode Island Change Assessment Scale

McConnaughy, DiClemente, Prochaska, and Velicer (McConnaughy, Prochaska, & Velicer, 1983; McConnaughy, DiClemente, Prochaska, & Velicer, 1989) developed the University of Rhode Island Change Assessment Scale (URICA) as a method of classifying subjects in stages of change when a straightforward algorithm does not work. The scale consists of 32 items that have been shown to reflect four stage of change factors: precontemplation, contemplation, action, and maintenance. The items describe attitudes, intentions, and behaviors associated with changing a target behavior. Furthermore, the URICA items are written generically, so they can apply to change in a range of behaviors. The stem or introduction to the items determines which specific behavior is the target of the assessment. Separate sets of eight items load on or are associated with each stage of change. Table 3.1 shows samples of items that are associated with each of the four stages of change included in the URICA.

In the area of substance abuse, the URICA has been used by specifying specific drugs (e.g., cocaine, marijuana, heroin, alcohol) or the more generic "illegal drugs" as the target. Some have instead substituted the specific problem substance in the actual items.

Each of the items is responded to according to degree of agreement: strongly disagree (score of 1), disagree (2), undecided (3), agree (4), and strongly agree (5). The items are scored in the "positive" direction for each stage, so that the higher the score a person receives for a stage, the "more" he or she endorses attitudes and behaviors particular to that stage. With eight items for each stage, the highest score a person can receive for a stage is 40 and the lowest is 8.

This brief introduction to the URICA shows that a person actually can be assigned a score for each of the stages of change. Such a method of scoring contrasts with the categorical approach to measurement of stage of change that involves assignment of a person to a discrete category of change. By receiving a score for each stage, individuals can be "clustered,"

TABLE 3.1. Two University of Rhode Island Change Assessment Scale (URICA) Items for Each of Four Stages of Change

Stage of change	Items
Precontemplation	• As far as I'm concerned, I don't have any problems that need changing. • I guess I have faults, but there's nothing I really need to change.
Contemplation	• I think I might be ready for some self-improvement. • I wish I had more ideas on how to solve my problem.
Action	• I am finally doing some work on my problem. • Anyone can talk about changing; I'm actually doing something about it.
Maintenance	• I'm not following through with what I had already changed as well as I had hoped, and I'm here to prevent a relapse of the problem. • I thought once I had resolved the problem I would be free of it, but sometimes I find myself struggling with it.

Note. When used in the assessment of substance use, the instructional set would indicate that the client should respond to the items in the context of their general drug use or in the context of a specific substance (e.g., cocaine, alcohol, heroin). Alternatively, the scale items themselves can be modified to reflect a particular substance (e.g., the action item "I am finally doing some work on my problem" could be revised to "I am finally doing some work on my cocaine problem").

or grouped, according to the pattern of scores on the four stage of change subscales (as described in Chapter 2). The clusters may be labeled either according to a "dominant" (according to score) stage of change or according to the researcher's or clinician's interpretation of what the pattern of subscale scores says about the person's attitudes toward or perceptions of changing the problem behavior. This latter method of interpreting a combination of scores contributed to the identification of the preparation "stage" (see Chapter 1). Research that has been completed with this clustering approach has revealed excellent consistency in subscale score patterns among, for example, inpatient and outpatient alcoholics and individuals receiving treatment at a weight loss clinic (Prochaska & DiClemente, 1992). Research on a sample of individuals presenting for outpatient alcohol treatment (Carbonari, DiClemente, Addy, & Pollack,

1996) has yielded alternative short forms of the URICA (two 12-item versions and a 24-item version). In addition, clinical researchers have been evaluating the use of a continuous "readiness to change" score that is calculated by summing the subscale scores for the contemplation, action, and maintenance stages and subtracting the precontemplation subscale score. This readiness score has been found to predict abstinence from drinking outcomes among outpatients receiving alcoholism treatment (DiClemente, Carbonari, Zweben, Morrel, & Lee, 2001; Project MATCH Research Group, 1997a).

In summary, the URICA has become the most common way of measuring stages of change. The scale allows for identification of individuals by the pattern of their subscale scores. These patterns or profiles have been named either according to a dominant stage of change score or by interpretation of a combination of scores. The profile approach so far has revealed excellent consistency in stage of change score patterns across diverse populations. With this as a basis, clusters may then be correlated with other variables that are of conceptual or clinical importance.

Stages of Change Readiness and Treatment Eagerness Scale

The Stages of Change Readiness and Treatment Eagerness Scale (SOCRATES) was developed by Miller and his colleagues (Miller & Tonigan, 1996) and is analogous to the URICA in concept, even using some of the same items. The SOCRATES consists of 40 items constructed and scored in a way similar to the URICA. Respondents indicate their degree of agreement with an item and accordingly can receive a score from 1 to 5. The scores for eight items then are summed to give a scale score for each of five stages of change, namely precontemplation, contemplation, preparation, action, and maintenance. In this sense the SOCRATES yields a profile of stage scores and, like the URICA, can be used to identify a person's "dominant" stage. Table 3.2 presents sample items that constitute each of the five SOCRATES-identified stages of change.

Miller and Tonigan (1996) reported the development of a 19-item short form of SOCRATES that has good psychometric properties and research and clinical utility. The 19 items that constitute the brief SOCRATES were selected from among the 40 items making up the longer form. Analyses of responses to the brief SOCRATES items by a sample of individuals presenting for alcohol treatment showed that the briefer

TABLE 3.2. Two Stages of Change Readiness and Treatment Eagerness Scale (SOCRATES) Items for Each of Five Stages of Change

Stage of change	Items
Precontemplation	• The only reason I'm here is that somebody made me come. • I am a fairly normal drinker.
Contemplation	• Sometimes I wonder if my drinking is hurting other people. • I don't think I have "a problem" with drinking, but there are times when I wonder if I drink too much.
Preparation	• I am a problem drinker. • I drink too much at times.
Action	• I have already been trying to change my drinking, and I am here to get some more help with it. • I have started to carry out a plan to cut down or stop my drinking.
Maintenance	• I am worried that my previous problems with drinking might come back. • Now that I have changed my drinking, it is important for me to hold onto the change I've made.

Note. Items may be adjusted to measure stage of change for drug use other than alcohol by substituting the drug(s) in question for references to drinking and alcohol.

measure taps into three dimensions, called Taking Steps (to change drinking behavior), Recognition (that the respondent has an alcohol problem), and Ambivalence (about whether the respondent has an alcohol problem). Miller and Tonigan (1996) have recommended use of the brief SOCRATES over the longer version of the instrument.

Readiness to Change Questionnaire

Rollnick, Heather, Gold, and Hall (1992) presented a questionnaire that also was based on Prochaska and DiClemente's ideas about stages of change and the URICA questionnaire. The Rollnick et al. scale, however, is briefer (12 items) than the URICA or SOCRATES. Like the SOC-

RATES, the Readiness to Change Questionnaire (RCQ) focuses on readiness to change drinking behavior. The scale originally was created for use with individuals who presented in a setting for treatment of medical problems.

The RCQ is composed of 12 items, clustered into three stages (each with four items) called precontemplation, contemplation, and action. Table 3.3 shows a sample of one item from each of the three stages.

Responses to each of the RCQ items can range from strongly disagree (score of −2), through 0, to strongly agree (score of +2). Therefore, for each stage of change a person's score can range from −8 to +8. As does the URICA, this scale places respondents on a continuum within each stage of change. Initial studies of the RCQ (Rollnick et al., 1992) show that it has good psychometric properties as well as the ability to predict treatment outcomes (Heather et al., 1993).

Progress has been excellent in validating the premise that people can be identified with a stage of change. Continued research will likely confirm the idea that, rather than a strict stage model of change, a combination of stage and continuum of readiness for change models will best describe individuals' preparedness for change (see, e.g., Miller & Tonigan, 1996). Despite the important and interesting questions about how to conceptualize a person's "location" in the change process, for ease of discussion and organization we will keep the discrete stage of change idea intact except where this simplifying approach misrepresents an idea or some information.

TABLE 3.3. Sample Items of the Readiness for Change Questionnaire Representing Each of Three Stages of Change

Stage of change	Sample item
Precontemplation	• It's a waste of time thinking about my drinking.
Contemplation	• I am at the stage where I should think about drinking less alcohol.
Action	• I am trying to drink less than I used to.

Note. Items may be adjusted to measure stage of change for drug use other than alcohol by substituting the drug(s) in question for references to drinking and alcohol.

ASSESSMENTS WITH PARTICULAR RELEVANCE TO CLIENTS IN THE PRECONTEMPLATION, CONTEMPLATION, AND PREPARATION STAGES

Among the measures most relevant to the assessment of persons in the precontemplation, contemplation, and preparation stages are those used for substance abuse screening and for the identification and specification of problem areas (including measures designed for purposes of assessing actual alcohol and drug use and for making diagnostic determinations). Such basic assessments have as a goal the defining of the nature and extent of the pattern of substance use in a way that is descriptive, shows its full functional properties, and leads to diagnostic conclusions. These assessments taken together can be used for two important functions. The first is to develop feedback for clients on their substance use and its consequences. This feedback is of clinical value generally, and perhaps especially to clients in the precontemplation and contemplation stages of change, because in these stages individuals either do not acknowledge a problem or are not firmly committed to changing it. The second important function of these assessments is to develop hypotheses about what factors are maintaining the person's pattern of alcohol and drug use, which has direct relevance to treatment planning.

With the above as preface, we review in the following sections the major biological and self-report measures for identifying individuals who have alcohol or other drug problems. We concentrate on breath test, urinalysis, and blood test procedures for biological methods, and on the interview and questionnaire for self-report methods.

Biological Methods

Breath Testing

The most common assessment for the presence of alcohol in the system is the breath test. The breath test is popular because it is noninvasive, accurate when correctly used, portable, inexpensive, and quick and easy to administer. Because of all of these advantages, there has been concerted effort to produce a similarly convenient way to measure for the presence of other drugs by breath test. Unfortunately, a satisfactory method has yet to be developed.

The major use of breath testing as a screening method is that it can serve as an indicator of possible alcohol problems that, if positive, would be followed up with additional assessment. For example, if an individual presented for an interview in some setting, or for some purpose other than substance abuse treatment, such as an appointment for medical care or for psychiatric care, the presence of alcohol in the person's system could be a sign of heavy drinking patterns and associated problems. A positive blood alcohol concentration then would be evaluated further by any of the various screening techniques that are described below.

Breath testing also can serve as an important clinical tool in treating individuals for their already identified problems with alcohol and drugs. For example, routine breath testing of individuals before beginning each of their treatment sessions may encourage their sobriety.

Urinalysis

Urinalysis probably is the most popular method of testing for the presence of drugs other than alcohol in the blood, although alcohol also can be detected by urinalysis. Urinalysis can, with cost differences, provide a qualitative (drug present or absent) or quantitative (how much drug, if it is present) measure of drug concentration. Urinalysis gives a measure of use over the past 2 to 3 days for most drugs of abuse, and over a week or longer in cases of heavy cannabis or phencyclidine use (Anton, Litton, & Allen, 1995; Schwartz, 1988).

Despite advancements in the use of urinalysis procedures over the past several decades (DeAngelis, 1971; Maisto, McKay, & Connors, 1990), there remain several major considerations in the use of urinalysis. This is particularly true because of the now widespread use of urinalysis in different settings. The first point to consider is the interpretation of any single test outcome. One true, positive outcome, for example, is not evidence for current drug intoxication or impairment, or of frequency and duration of drug use. In this regard, individual user differences in the potency of drug used, in the administration of the drug, and in the rates of drug absorption, distribution, and metabolism, as well as actual use, may affect a true positive finding. As a result, drawing conclusions from just one test is not good practice.

Another concern is the problem of false positive and false negative findings. A false positive result can occur by "confusing" the analytical method. For example, an individual may use a legal substance that imitates some drug of abuse, which would result in a positive finding for the drug of abuse. A false negative finding usually is the more common concern of people doing the testing. Such findings often occur through the user's deliberate efforts to invalidate a test, such as by using a nonuser's urine sample or by adulterating the urine sample to interfere with its analysis. A false negative finding also may result from the tester's failure to appreciate the span of time of previous drug use that urinalysis can detect. For example, a person may have used cocaine daily and heavily for up to 6 days before urinalysis. And, in response to the question "How much cocaine have you used in the past week?," the user may reply, "None." The urine test would corroborate the "none" response.

In summary, urinalysis can be an accurate tool for identifying and following up with individuals with alcohol or drug problems. However, its value depends on following well-specified procedures in its use.

Blood Tests

The methods we have described so far all are ways to detect the presence of alcohol or other drugs in the blood and thus are measures of recent use. Of course, blood samples can be analyzed directly for this same purpose. However, blood samples also can be analyzed for evidence of longer-term (recent weeks to years) heavy alcohol use. This can be done, first, by testing for elevation of liver enzymes, which is correlated with heavy alcohol consumption in the past month. The tests in this category that are used commonly include aspartate aminotransferase (AST), alanine aminotransferase (ALT), and gamma-glutamyltransferase (GGT) (e.g., Anton et al., 1995; Niles & McCrady, 1991). Another test for alteration in blood cells, called mean cell volume (MCV), also can be used to test for recent heavy drinking.

All four of these tests may be significantly elevated (compared to the normal range values) with past heavy drinking. GGT is the most sensitive of the tests to changes (whether increases or decreases) in alcohol consumption (Anton et al., 1995). Although these blood tests have received the most attention as screening and identification methods, particularly in medical settings, they also often are used in the treatment and evaluation of individuals already identified as having alcohol problems.

A test for GGT, AST, ALT, or MCV should not be used alone as a screening method for several reasons (Leigh & Skinner, 1988). First, the test may be affected by using drugs other than alcohol, so there is not excellent specificity (for alcohol) of these biochemical tests. This is a problem not only for what are typically called the drugs of "abuse"; for example, MCV may be elevated by cigarette smoking. Another problem is that when the person tested is in good physical health, the test is far less likely to be elevated even if recent heavy drinking did occur. Relatedly, the tests have good specificity in general population studies but do less well in discriminating between alcoholics and medically ill nonalcoholics (Anton et al., 1995). This is because test values may be elevated by disease processes that have little to do with high alcohol use. Third, the degree of elevation of the tests and quantity of alcohol consumed does not follow a simple linear pattern. So, for example, as quantity of alcohol increases, enzyme elevation does not increase proportionately throughout the range of values that are possible. Therefore, the relationship between alcohol consumption and blood test score is complex. Relatedly, there are large differences among individuals in the relationship between alcohol use and lab test scores. Finally, lab test scores alone may discriminate most productively between individuals who are light, nonproblem drinkers and those who already have suffered serious consequences from heavy alcohol use. However, even groups of laboratory tests do a poor job in identifying individuals with mild to moderate impairment due to alcohol (Watson, Mohs, Eskelson, Sampliner, & Hartmann, 1986). A good screening method should be able to identify cases with less severe alcohol problems.

These problems should not be taken to imply that biochemical measures of recent heavy drinking should be discarded altogether. Rather, the weaknesses of the tests point up the necessity of using them in conjunction with other measures. In this regard, relevant recommendations have included using combinations of laboratory tests (Leigh & Skinner, 1988) and using laboratory tests with such measures as screening questionnaires and a client's clinical record (Anton et al., 1995; Babor, Kranzler, & Lauerman, 1989; Niles & McCrady, 1991; Leigh & Skinner, 1988).

Self-Report Screening Methods

Screening methods that involve responding to questions from an interviewer or to items on a questionnaire about the use of alcohol and associated consequences are well established and researched for the detection of alcohol problems. However, there are far fewer measures available for the identification of individuals with other drug problems. Although several instruments have the stated purpose of identifying drug abuse in adults, all but one (the Drug Abuse Screening Test, reviewed below) are too long to be of practical value in most clinical settings. In this section we review the most important and widely used self-report alcohol and drug use disorder screening measures.

Michigan Alcoholism Screening Test

The Michigan Alcoholism Screening Test (MAST) was developed by Selzer (1971) in order to provide a quick, systematic, quantifiable way to "diagnose" alcoholism that could be administered by professionals and paraprofessionals alike. In fact, the MAST more accurately is seen today as a method that helps to identify—not to diagnose—individuals with alcohol problems.

The original MAST consists of 25 items relating to primarily negative consequences (whether physical, psychological, family, or legal) of alcohol use. Each item is answered by checking "Yes" or "No." Items are weighted, which means that responses to some items suggesting the presence of alcohol use disorder receive more points (in a range of 1 to 5) than do other responses. A total score of 0 to 53 is possible, with a score of 5 or higher suggestive of alcoholism. The MAST can be self-administered, taking about 5 to 10 minutes, or it can be administered by an interviewer, which takes about 15 to 20 minutes (Jacobson, 1989). Examples of MAST items are "Do you feel you are a normal drinker?"; "Have you ever lost a job because of drinking?"; and "Have you ever gotten into trouble at work because of your drinking?"

It is obvious from the foregoing sample items that the MAST "pulls" for problems with alcohol. Depending on whether the testing situation encourages or discourages accurate reporting of consequences related to alcohol use, this has led to an over- or underidentification of alcoholism. Jacobson's (1989) summary of the large volume of research on the MAST suggests, however, that maintaining a cutoff score of 5 overidentifies. He advises adjusting the cutoff score to as high as 12, depending on preference for a test more sensitive in identifying alcoholics or a test that is better at specifying a person who does not have problems with alcohol.

One feature of the MAST is important to discuss because it may contribute to overidentification of individuals as having current alcohol problems. The sample MAST items we listed above show there is a lack of a consistent time referent for the items: Some items refer to current status ("Do you feel you are a normal drinker?"), while others refer to a lifetime ("Have you ever gotten into trouble at work because of your drinking?"). Therefore, if the interest is in identifying people with current alcohol problems only, this lack of a consistent time referent would tend to result in a higher number of false positives. One way around this problem, if the MAST is administered by an interviewer, is to ask the respondent "when?" if he or she answers a "lifetime referent" test item in the direction of alcoholism (see Jacobson, 1989).

The great popularity of the MAST led to two briefer versions, the 13-item Short Michigan Alcoholism Screening Test (SMAST) and the 10-item Brief Michigan Alcoholism Screening Test (BMAST) (Selzer, Vinokur, & van Rooijen, 1975, and Pokorny, Miller, & Kaplan, 1972, respectively). The Self-Administered Michigan Alcoholism Screening Test (Swenson & Morse, 1975) is another MAST derivative. Jacobson (1989) argues that these MAST modifications have "reasonable" reliability and validity, but Gibbs's (1983) review suggests that the MAST is more reliable. These comments notwithstanding, the high face validity (or obviousness) of the MAST and its derivatives suggests that the degree of validity may closely reflect the context of test administration.

Drug Abuse Screening Test

As the acronym suggests, the Drug Abuse Screening Test (DAST) is the MAST counterpart for problems with drugs other than alcohol. This test was developed by Skinner (1982), and the original version consisted of 28 items that are answered "Yes" or "No." The current version of the DAST includes the 20 items that discriminated criterion groups most productively in validation studies. Analogous to the MAST, the DAST primarily focuses on the consequences of drug use and can be self-administered or administered by an interviewer. The DAST is also analogous to the MAST in the inconsistent time references of the DAST's 20 items. Some examples include "Have you used drugs other than those required for medical reasons?"; "Do you abuse more than one drug at a time?"; and "Does your spouse (or parents) ever complain about your involvement with drugs?"

The DAST items are not assigned any weights, so that a person's score for the test is the simple sum of the number of items answered in the direction of increased drug problems. Therefore, scores can range from 0 to 20. Unlike the MAST, no formally developed cutoff scores (for identifying persons with drug problems) are available. However, the initial validation study of the DAST that Skinner (1982) completed suggests that scores of 6 or higher are indicative of drug problems. Furthermore, as DAST scores increase, the implication is that the individual's drug problems are more severe (see Babor, 1993). At present, the DAST is best viewed as one of the few screening tests for drug abuse that are based on good research, but also as a test that is in need of additional evaluation.

CAGE

The CAGE (Mayfield, McLeod, & Hall, 1974) is the briefest of the self-report screening methods that we have presented so far. The test name is an acronym of letters of words in the only four items that make up the test: (1) "Have you ever felt you should Cut down on your drinking?"; (2) "Have people Annoyed you by criticizing your drinking?"; (3) "Have you ever felt Guilty about your drinking?"; and (4) "Have you ever had a drink first thing in the morning (Eye opener)?" These four questions are asked by an interviewer, taking only a few minutes at most. A cutoff score of 2 to 3 items answered "Yes" seems to work most productively for sensitive and accurate identification (Jacobson, 1989).

There are a couple of points that are important to note in using the CAGE. The first is that the high face validity and the paucity of items suggest that if a positive identification is made it should be corroborated, if at all possible, by another data source, such as the respondent's spouse. In this regard, such a practice has become common in using the MAST and derivatives because of their obvious intent. The second point is that the CAGE questions have no time referent, so that, for example, an item could be answered positively because of events of 20 years ago but not currently. This suggests that, in some cases, the CAGE would yield too many positives in relation to *current* alcohol problems. As we noted in our discussion of the MAST, Jacobson (1989) suggests one way to solve this problem is to ask "when" or for more information for any question that is answered yes.

A method that Cyr and Wartman (1988) reported beats the brevity of the CAGE by two items in identifying alcohol problems. This study involved case identification of men and women who were admitted to a primary care unit of a large teaching hospital in southern New England. While the clients were waiting for their first appointment with their new physicians, they were interviewed for about 45 minutes regarding medical history, family history (for alcohol problems), health habits, and alcohol use. Essentially, the idea was to cover screening for alcoholism, risk factors for alcoholism, and standard alcohol history. After the interview was completed, a research assistant administered the MAST.

Cyr and Wartman used all the information they collected to see what interview information they collected predicted a "diagnosis" of alcoholism, as determined by MAST score (cutoff score of 5). It was found that two interview questions, "Have you ever had a drinking problem?" and "When was your last drink?" (a response of within the last 24 hours should be considered a positive indicator), together were excellent predictors of a positive identification on the MAST. A total of 91.5% of the MAST alcoholics answered one or both of these questions positively, while 89.7% of the MAST nonalcoholics answered negatively to one or both questions. This test performance outdistanced by far the predictive value of other interview questions, such as "How much do you drink?" and "How often do you drink?"

These findings attracted a lot of attention because of the idea that it is possible to identify alcohol problems in a primary medical care setting with such a quick, efficient method, even beating out the CAGE. Of course, there are caveats before getting swept away by the results. For example, the diagnostic criterion used in the study (MAST score) is tenuous, and both the MAST and the interview items are highly face valid and have no time boundaries. In this regard, a person could answer positively to the "problems" items on both the MAST and the Cyr and Wartman questions but have no current alcohol problems, since both the latter questions and the MAST have open-ended time references. Also, whether the results can be repeated with other samples and settings is still open to research. Yet, the implications of this study should be most appealing to case finders.

Alcohol Use Disorders Identification Test

The Cyr and Wartman (1988) study leads to discussion of the Alcohol Use Disorders Identification Test (AUDIT), which is a 10-item screening measure that was designed specifically for use in the medical treatment setting. In particular, the AUDIT was developed for use in primary care clinics, although research shows that it is suited for use in other settings as well, such as psychiatric clinics, the legal system, and the military (Allen & Columbus, 1995; Saunders, Aasland, Babor, de la Fuente, & Grant, 1993).

The response to each of the 10 items of the AUDIT is given a score, and the total score is derived simply by adding the individual's score for each of the respective items. The minimum (cutoff) score for possible indication of alcohol problems is 8. Administration of the test takes only a few minutes, and its scoring even takes less time than that. Furthermore, research strongly supports the AUDIT's reliability and validity (Connors, 1995). In brief, the AUDIT is a more recently developed screening measure that is becoming increasingly popular because of its ease of administration and scoring, applicability to several different case-finding settings, and research support for its reliability and validity.

MacAndrew Scale

So far we have reviewed self-report methods of identification that are obvious in what they are designed to measure. The MacAndrew Scale (MAC) stands in stark contrast to these in that it has low face validity, that is, is not so obvious (given the questions). This scale, which was developed by MacAndrew (1965), has no items pertaining to alcohol, its use, or consequences related to its use. Instead, the MAC consists of 49 items from the Minnesota Multiphasic Personality Inventory (MMPI) that have been shown to discriminate empirically between alcoholics and other groups. The MAC is self-administered, and respondents answer "true" or "false" to each item. The test takes about 15 minutes to complete.

Jacobson (1989) reports that the MAC is sensitive to identifying people who actually have alcohol problems, but it also falsely identifies others as positive for alcohol problems who actually are not. These groups include nonalcoholic drug users, heavy cigarette smokers, and heavy users of caffeine. This implies that if a positive MAC score is obtained it should be corroborated by another data source. Jacobson suggests these cutoff scores for the MAC: < 23, negative; 24–27, possible; > 28, positive (Jacobson, 1989, p. 25).

During the 1980s the MMPI was revised, and in 1989 the MMPI-2 was published (Graham, 1999). The MAC scale is retained in the MMPI-2, with the same number of items, and is called the MAC-R(evised). The only difference between the MAC-R and the MAC is that four MAC items were replaced with four other items that discriminate between individuals who have alcohol problems and those who do not. Therefore, scores on the MAC-R may be interpreted similarly to scores on the MAC (Graham, 1999).

To summarize this section, research has produced several self-report alcohol screening questionnaires that are brief, inexpensive, and easy to administer in virtually any clinical setting. Unfortunately, practical screening instruments that focus on other drugs of abuse are not nearly so common.

It is important to note that the goals and the context of the screening may affect which measure is selected. For example, Connors's (1995) review shows that in studies directly comparing the two instruments the MAST tends to be more sensitive than the CAGE but that the CAGE may perform better than the MAST with elderly primary care clients.

Intake Interview and Structured Diagnostic Interview Schedules

Intake Interview

The mainstay measure of almost all substance abuse treatment programs is the personal intake interview. The common core across all intake interviews is questions regarding substance use history, patterns, and consequences, although the specific format and content of such interviews vary considerably from one treatment program to another.

Questions about substance use history generally emphasize onset of use, perceived years of problem use of alcohol or other drugs, context of substance use, reasons for substance use, family history of alcohol or other drug problems, patterns of substance use, and quantity and frequency of alcohol and other drug use. Questions on consequences of substance use usually emphasize the domains of physical and psychological health, social and marital/family relationships, job performance, and legal factors (especially arrests related to substance use, such as driving under the influence).

One important area of questioning in intake interviews is symptoms of physical dependence on alcohol or other drugs. For example, for alcohol, questions might be asked about current or lifetime occurrence of hangovers, shakes (tremors), seizures or convulsions, "loss of control" drinking, hallucinations, delirium tremens, memory impairment and blackouts, tolerance, and drinking to quell withdrawal symptoms. Finally, intake interviews often include inquiries about past attempts to resolve substance use problems, such as efforts to reduce use without the help of formal treatment, attendance at self-help groups (e.g., Alcoholics Anonymous, Narcotics Anonymous), or the use of formal treatment.

The intake interview is the source of information that is used in the vast majority of substance abuse treatment settings as the main source of diagnosis. Because they tend to reflect the treatment philosophy of a program staff and any idiosyncratic needs of a program, clinical intake interviews generally are characterized by their lack of standardization in interview content, format, and administration. The result is that it is impossible to compare with any faith intake data for different treatment settings or even for different respondents in the same treatment settings.

One obvious way around this difficulty is to standardize. An example of such an intake interview is Miller and Marlatt's (1984) Comprehensive Drinker Profile (CDP). The CDP was designed to enable systematic collection of data on the use of alcohol and on other areas of life functioning, including other drug use. Part of what makes the CDP standardized is that it is accompanied by a manual to guide interview administration and interpretation of responses. The CDP earns the "comprehensive" part of its name, as it includes questions on client demographics, family and living situation, employment, education, drinking history (including development of the alcohol problem, current drinking pattern, and alcohol-related problems), other substance use, medical and psychiatric history, and motivation for treatment. The CDP takes about 50 minutes to administer. If a shorter interview is desired, the Brief Drinker Profile also is available.

Structured Diagnostic Interview Schedules

These measures may be viewed as "specialized" intake interviews, as they are geared specifically to collecting data for the purpose of categorization in a system of psychiatric nomenclature. Formal diagnosis may be of considerable help in treatment planning, and it is generally required in any case in accredited substance abuse treatment settings. The advantage in the use of formal measures in arriving at diagnosis is the same as we described in discussing the CDP, namely, a better opportunity for reliability and validity in the information gathered. We include formal diagnosis in this section of the chapter (as opposed to the following section on action and maintenance) because diagnosis is potentially relevant to case identification, as selected diagnostic instruments have been designed for evaluating individuals who might appear outside the substance abuse treatment setting.

The four instruments that we present in this section pertain to diagnosis of substance use disorders as well as other adult psychopathology. The instruments originally were developed primarily for epidemiological and clinical research purposes but often are used clinically to the benefit of treatment planning. They take about 60 to 90 minutes to administer in their entirety. Naturally, just administering sections on substance use can take considerably less time. Times for administration vary with the respondent, as "skip options" are available if the respondent "screens out" of any disorder. Furthermore, interviews may be administered in person or by computer.

Table 3.4 provides some specific details about four diagnostic interviews commonly used by substance abuse clinicians and researchers: the Diagnostic Interview Schedule (DIS); the Structured Clinical Interview for DSM-IV (SCID); the SCID Alcohol/Drug Version (SCID-A/D); and the Alcohol Use Disorders and Associated Disabilities Interview Schedule (AUDADIS). Using the information in Table 3.4 to compare the instruments shows that choice of a diagnostic measure depends on the answers to questions about purpose of making diagnoses, characteristics of interviewers and respondents, resources for staff training, and requirements for reliability and validity. Much more detail is available on each of the instruments listed in Table 3.4 by writing to different sources on the measures (contact information is provided in Hasin, 1991, p. 299, and Allen & Columbus, 1995).

Multivariate Measures

Many excellent measures of single variables or factors that are relevant to assessment in substance abuse treatment settings have been developed. For example, single-variable measures concern only one construct, such as expectations about alcohol and drug effects, self-esteem, or social support. Because of the large number and variety of single-variable measures in the substance abuse treatment area, we will not attempt to review them here; several reviews are available for the interested reader (e.g., Allen & Columbus, 1995; Donovan & Marlatt, 1988; Maisto & Connors, 1990). For our purposes, the listing in Table 3.5 of recommended areas of measurement of individuals presenting for drug or alcohol treatment gives a good idea of the number of single-factor measures that are available, given that most areas of assessment have many such measures associated with them.

In keeping with our emphasis on multivariate models of substance abuse, we will discuss two self-report measures that are designed to cap-

TABLE 3.4. Major Standardized Diagnostic Instruments

Instrument	Main features	Training required for administration
Diagnostic Interview Schedule (DIS)	• Fully structured, designed for administration by nonclinicians • Newer version linked to DSM-IV criteria	• Read manual, complete homework assignments, attend 1-week training session.
Structured Clinical Interview for DSM-IV (SCID)	• Semistructured, designed for use by experienced clinical interviewers • Linked to DSM-IV criteria	• Read brief user's guide, watch 6-hour videotape. Option of SCID trainer visit to training site (interviewers assumed to be already experienced and knowledgeable in clinical interviewing).
SCID Alcohol/ Drug Version (SCID-A/D)	• Semistructured, based on standard SCID but more structured • Differs from standard SCID in emphasis on reliable assessment of community residents (thus milder symptoms) as well as patients • As with standard SCID, interviewers must have clinical skills and knowledge of diagnostic criteria	• More extensive and formal than standard SCID. Include study of SCID/AD training manual, completion of self-study questions, rating of videotaped interviews, 4 days of role playing and lectures on the SCID/AD, watching and rating additional videotaped interviews, further role playing with trainers, audiotaping own interview for review by trainers.
Alcohol Use Disorders and Associated Disabilities Interview Schedule (AUDADIS)	• Fully structured, designed for use by nonclinicians • Also may be used in clinical settings • Linked to criteria of DSM-III-R; for alcohol and other drug diagnoses, uses criteria of DSM-III, ICD-10, and DSM IV • Allows assessment of symptoms over a broad range of severities • Especially good for evaluating relationship between substance use and other psychiatric disorders • Must be administered in person	• Use of self-study materials, 5 days of classroom training, and completion of trainer-observed interviews.

Note. Data from Hasin (1991).

TABLE 3.5. Recommended Areas to Assess in Individuals Presenting for Treatment of Alcohol or Other Drug Problems

- Specific quantities of alcohol or other drugs used, and the frequency of their use
- Predominant mood states and situations antecedent and consequent to substance use
- Usual and unusual substance use circumstances and patterns
- History of alcohol and other drug withdrawal symptoms
- Medical problems associated with or exacerbated by substance use
- Identification of possible difficulties the patient may have in initially refraining from substance use
- Extent and severity of previous substance use problems
- Multiple drug use
- Reports of frequent thoughts or urges to drink or take drugs
- History of previous responses to alcohol or drug treatment and self-initiated periods of abstinence
- Review of the positive consequences of substance use
- Other life problems
- Indicants of tolerance to alcohol or other drugs
- Past or present indicants of liver disorder
- (For alcohol use) Risks associated with considering a nonabstinent treatment goal

Note. Adapted from Sobell, Sobell, and Nirenberg (1988, pp. 23–26); Sobell, Toneatto, and Sobell (1994); and Maisto, O'Farrell, Worthen, and Walitzer (1993).

ture multiple dimensions of substance use and related problems. These are the Alcohol Use Inventory and the Addiction Severity Index.

Alcohol Use Inventory

The Alcohol Use Inventory (AUI; Horn et al., 1987; Wanberg, Horn, & Foster, 1977) is a 228-item test that was developed to measure multiple features of alcohol use and consequences in individuals presenting for treatment of alcohol problems. The items, which are presented in a multiple-choice format, reflect 24 scales, or factors. The test takes about 35 minutes to complete and can be computer or hand scored.

The 24 AUI scales were derived through extensive research. The scales reflect the respondent's style of alcohol use, the benefits he or she perceives to receive from drinking, negative consequences of drinking, and awareness that the respondent has about his or her alcohol problem and concerns about it. Note that this last area of evaluation, which actually is one scale of the AUI, fits nicely as a precontemplation/contemplation stage measure, as it is directly relevant to the central questions of those stages of change.

One of the outstanding features of the AUI that warrants mention is that it can be used to match individuals to specific treatment settings (e.g., inpatient or outpatient) or to treatment modalities (e.g., individual or family). Therefore, the AUI is one of the few assessments available in the substance abuse area that take direct steps toward being treatment prescriptive. In the user's guide for the AUI (Horn et al., 1987), the authors discuss how the test results can be used for specific, individualized treatment planning. An excellent example of how AUI data can be used to identify "profiles" of alcohol abusing clients was recently provided by Rychtarik, Koutsky, and Miller (1998, 1999).

In summary, the AUI is a well-developed, well-evaluated, and clinically valuable multivariate measure of alcohol use and related consequences. Full appreciation of the AUI's development, content, and use can be obtained by study of the test guide (Horn et al., 1987). Currently it is one of the most useful multivariate measures available for individuals who present for alcohol treatment.

Addiction Severity Index

In contrast to the AUI, the Addiction Severity Index (ASI) was designed for use with individuals who present for alcohol or other drug treatment. The ASI is a structured personal interview that was designed to measure the severity of problems in five different areas that are typically affected as part of individuals' alcohol or other drug abuse: medical, employment, legal, family relations, and psychiatric. Severity of both alcohol and other drug use also is measured. The ASI was developed for use in treatment planning upon clients' admission to treatment and as a measure of change during and following treatment (McLellan et al., 1992; McLellan, Luborsky, Woody, & O'Brien, 1980).

In each of the seven areas of functioning that is measured with the ASI, questions are asked on the number, frequency, and duration of the problem symptoms, both in a client's lifetime and in the past 30 days. From these basic data, two different scores are derived. First, the individual receives a composite score in each area based on answers given to each of the items that constitutes an area of functioning. These scores reflect problem area severity and are arithmetically derived from key interview items comprising each area. Clients' perceptions of problem severity also are obtained for each area by asking them to rate both the severity of the problem and their need of further treatment for it. Lastly, after the interview is completed, the interviewer is asked to judge the severity of each problem area by rating the need for further treatment, based on responses to individual items and on the client's perception of need for treatment and how troubled he or she is by the problem in question.

Since the ASI was published in 1980, it has become a popular instrument in alcohol and drug treatment settings in the United States, Canada, and Europe. In general, reliability and validity data are good, and they hold up across different client populations defined by age, sex, race, and primary drug problem. In addition, the psychometric properties of the ASI have been shown to be sound when evaluated in several European nations. However, the psychometric properties of the interviewer severity ratings have been found to be more variable across the problem areas (Alterman, Brown, Zaballero, & McKay, 1994).

The ASI takes about 50 to 60 minutes to complete by a competent interviewer. Requirements for learning to give the ASI are minimal, with the ability to communicate effectively with people who present for substance abuse treatment the basic necessity. Training is possible through use of an on-site training package that is available from the test developers.

To summarize, the ASI is a multivariate measure of severity of substance use and related areas of functioning. It is an excellent measure to use for assessment of individuals who present for alcohol or other drug treatment and can be an important part of feedback development and treatment planning.

Measures of Alcohol and Other Drug Use

Alcohol Consumption

The desired features of a measure of alcohol use are that it provide reliable, valid, and precise information on quantity of use, frequency of use, and patterns of use over specified time periods. Such time periods typically range from 30 days to 1 year before treatment admission. This collection of desirable measure features, along with a specified time period of at least 30 days, would allow for measurement of alcohol use that would be most helpful in treatment planning and that would enable sensitive measurement of changes in drinking during treatment and following its termination.

In the area of alcohol research and treatment many and varied measures of alcohol use have been developed. For clinical use, one measure has emerged that has our set of desirable features is the Timeline Followback (TLFB) interview (Sobell, Maisto, Sobell, & Cooper, 1979; Sobell & Sobell, 1992, 1996). In the TLFB interview, respondents are given a calendar and asked to provide estimates of their daily alcohol consumption over a given period of time. Research on the TLFB has included study of intervals of up to 360 days before the interview day. Respondents are helped in their recall of daily drinking by the use of memory aids, including the use of a visual calendar; the listing of key dates (holidays, birthdays, and so forth) on the calendar; the use of a standard drink conversion card (i.e., the quantities consumed of different alcoholic beverages are converted to "standard drinks"); and the identification of extended periods of drinking certain amounts, including no drinking.

Often the first reaction of interviewers and interviewees alike is that obtaining reasonable estimates of daily drinking for as far back as 1 year is pure fantasy. However, with only a minimum of training it becomes clear to new interviewers that such data can be reliably gathered. This has been demonstrated by the TLFB's impressive track record of successful use in both clinical and research settings since its publication in 1979.

Essentially, the scores that are derived from the daily drinking TLFB protocol are summary (over some period of time) indices. These may include, for example, percentage of days engaging in a given level or quantity of drinking, such as abstinence or heavy drinking days, maximum number of drinks on a day, or average number of drinks a day. In addition, information about temporal patterns in drinking can be derived (e.g., weekend, daily, or binge drinker). In effect, the initial collection of daily drinking data makes possible the use of a wide variety of summary variables that are specifically suited to the clinician's or researcher's needs.

Since the TLFB's appearance, research on its reliability and validity has been published extensively by both its developers and others. The data are consistently good in this regard, across different treatment settings and populations. Moreover, recently (Sobell & Sobell, 1996) the TLFB has become even more accessible with the publication of a manual that describes the TLFB's development and instructions for its administration, a training video, and software for computer administration of the TLFB. It is important to emphasize, however, that TLFB data are psychometrically sound only for the summary variables that we referenced earlier. Therefore, single-day estimates of drinking do not have research evidence to support their reliability and validity; as we discuss later, given the limitations of memory, such precision in retrospective measures probably should not be expected.

Form 90 Family of Instruments

As part of the design of the multiple site treatment-matching study called Project MATCH (Project MATCH Research Group, 1997a), the strengths of the TLFB and the alcohol consumption section of the Comprehensive Drinker Profile (described earlier in this chapter) were combined to create a new measure of alcohol consumption called the Form 90 (Miller & DelBoca, 1994). (The "family of instruments" refers to the multiple versions of Form 90, suited to different research or clinical needs, that are available.) Like the TLFB, the Form 90 is a structured interview that has the goal of recording retrospective self-reports of daily alcohol use. As its name implies, Form 90 is designed to collect information about the past 90 days. It yields information that is highly similar to that of the TLFB, but adds the ability to estimate what blood alcohol concentrations the individual reached on his or her drinking days. (Of course, making such estimates requires that the interviewer also obtain information from the respondent about the time course of alcohol consumption events.) Other differences between the TLFB and Form 90 primarily involve methods of administration to allow more efficient data collection when repetitive patterns and episodes of drinking are apparent in the respondent's drinking behavior. Psychometric assessments of the Form 90 have been positive (Tonigan, Miller, & Brown, 1997). As with the TLFB, a manual for the Form 90 is available (Miller, 1996), as is supporting computer software.

Other Drug Use

In discussing measurement of different variables relevant to substance abuse treatment, we have presented actual measures. However, in this section of self-report measures of consumption of drugs other than alcohol, we make an exception to that. As we discuss later, although there are examples of comprehensive measures of drug use, none is widely accepted. For this and other reasons that will become apparent in our discussion, we will not present examples of measures. It would seem to be more useful to review briefly the nuances and problems in measuring drug use, as well as to make recommendations in doing so. Clinicians then may apply these recommendations to their own assessment needs.

The desired features of a self-report measure of drug use are the same as those we listed for alcohol, with the addition of the need to measure route of administration of the drug and the combined use of more than one drug. Unfortunately, there are complexities in getting accurate information on drug use from an individual and in interpreting the information that is obtained that are not problems in measuring alcohol consumption (Maisto, McKay, & Connors, 1990; Martin & Wilkinson, 1989). These difficulties include, first, that sometimes it may be impossible to obtain data on quantities of street drugs sold, because often users do not know how much pharmacologically active ingredients are in the drugs they buy, and sometimes do not even know what drug they are buying. A second problem is in interpreting the data when multiple drugs are used: How should the data be combined to arrive at a single "drug use index"? It is no problem to combine the alcohol consumed in beer, wine, and hard liquor, because alcohol is common to the three types of beverages. But it is another matter to arrive at an analogous total use index for other drug use. The question is important, because a total use index would provide a quantitative statement about pretreatment drug use and would be a reference for measuring change from that level. Fortunately, there have been attempts to derive indices of total drug use, and we discuss these below. A last point also concerns interpretation of multiple drug use, including alcohol. In this regard, use of different drugs should not be seen as independent behaviors. Drugs may interact pharmacologically, resulting in an alteration of effects that are experienced by a given drug that may be different than what is experienced when that drug is taken alone. Also, behaviorally the use of one drug may be the antecedent or subsequent event of using another. For example, individuals may not use cocaine unless they already have drunk a certain amount of alcohol. Or, alcohol may be consumed following cocaine use to attenuate cocaine's stimulant effects.

Because of these and other complexities, methods of measuring drug use are far behind those in measuring alcohol use. Nevertheless, research has provided three guidelines for measuring drug consumption. These have been summarized by a task force in Ontario, Canada, that had the goal of developing a directory of measures of treatment outcome (Addiction Research Foundation, 1993). These principles are, first, to avoid using broad categories for drugs that are used frequently in the population of interest. Because there is no single generally accepted way to classify drugs, categorizations of them may be arbitrary. It is important to keep in mind that when categories are broad there may be differences of importance among drugs within a category, both in pharmacology and psychological and physical effects, as well as the problems that may result from use. Therefore, if a class of drugs is of major interest to the clinician or researcher, it is necessary to measure each drug as specifically as possible. It always is possible to form larger classifications later but difficult to do the reverse.

Another guideline in measurement is first to obtain information on the frequency of drug use. As we noted, accurate information on quantity of drug use may be difficult or impossible to obtain. Finally, besides frequency and, possibly, quantity information, it is important to obtain data on information such as route of administration, patterns of use, and the use of prescription medications.

It is fortunate that there have been a few good drug use measures developed for obtaining accurate data on lifetime and current street and prescription drug use. Illustrations of many of the most useful measures are provided in Addiction Research Foundation (1993). In addition, the TLFB and Form 90 may be used to collect information (primarily frequency data) on drug use other than alcohol (e.g., Ehrman & Robins, 1994; Fals-Stewart, O'Farrell, Freitas, McFarlin, & Rutigliano, 2000). These or other available drug use measures should be reviewed carefully before selecting one, with the idea of choosing the one that most productively addresses the clinical or research questions at hand for a given client population.

Once a measure of drug use is selected, there are somewhat different paths to follow for evaluation of single and multiple drug use. These paths are summarized in Figure 3.1. The problem is relatively simple when single drug use is the problem. In that case, with the use of structured and standardized interviews, there is little difficulty in collecting information on drug use frequency and route of administration. Once such data are obtained, they can be interpreted in a straightforward way. Furthermore, it then will be possible to measure change, say, in frequency of use over time. If it is possible to obtain accurate information on quantity of use, those data should be obtained as well, as a "bonus." The problem for multiple drug use differs because there is the need to obtain a drug use summary index so that a quantitative reference of change is available. As we explained, no generally accepted summary index has been developed, so

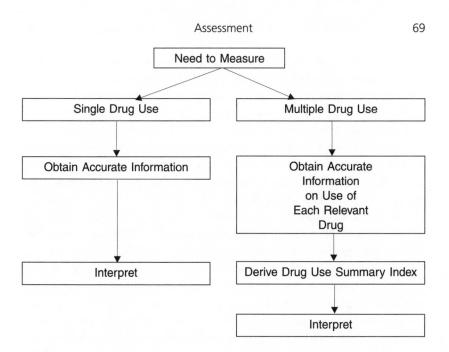

FIGURE 3.1. Flow chart of procedures to follow in measuring and interpreting single and multiple drug use.

the goal is to find or derive one that most productively suits the clinician's or researcher's specific needs. There are some examples in the literature, such as in Hubbard et al. (1989) and Wilkinson and LeBreton (1986).

To conclude our discussion of measuring drug use, no single standard self-report measure exists. It is unlikely that one will emerge any time soon, as patterns of drug use vary widely and are complex, drugs come and go and return again in popularity or availability, and different populations use different drugs differently (for example, compare the use of prescription drugs by adolescents and the elderly). For now, clinicians will need to obtain the information that is needed for a specific setting and purpose as accurately as possible and then interpret the data in a way that makes the most sense for the population in question.

Self-Monitoring: Self-Report of Current Behavior

Self-monitoring typically focuses on information for a behavioral assessment of current substance use, such as antecedents to use, frequency of use, patterns of use, and consequences of use. In self-monitoring, these data are not obtained by direct observation but by the person's monitoring and self-report of what is happening in his or her natural environment (e.g., Lemmens, Tan, & Knibbe, 1992; Sobell, Bogardis, Schuller, Leo, & Sobell, 1989).

When done properly, that is, the behavior is recorded when it occurs or at latest at the end of the day of occurrence, self-monitoring avoids the memory problems inherent in retrospective self-report methods of consumption such as the TLFB. And self-monitoring data are far more detailed than data collected when using retrospective measures. As such, self-monitoring provides an excellent assessment tool. It also is an excellent method to use in evaluating ongoing substance abuse treatment (e.g., Sobell, Toneatto, & Sobell, 1994). There are a few drawbacks to self-monitoring, however. The currency of the data is bought at the expense of obtaining information on longer-term past use. Therefore, self-monitoring obviously is not the method of choice when the interest is in learning about a client's substance use in the past 6 months. Another problem with self-monitoring is getting clients, or research subjects for that matter, to comply consistently with the request that they provide information about current substance use.

Summary

The large majority of clinical measures that have been developed in the alcohol and drug fields, including those discussed above, have been designed to obtain a better description and understanding of individuals, whether done briefly and efficiently in the context of screening or in greater detail with clients seeking treatment. In either case, the information gathered will be available for application in providing feedback to individuals about their alcohol and/or substance use and in the development of treatment plans for those seeking clinical services.

As noted earlier in this chapter, the provision of feedback to individuals based on assessment instruments such as those identified above is perhaps best exemplified in work with precontemplators and contemplators. Precontemplators are often characterized as having a lack of awareness of a problem and contemplators as struggling with the pros and cons of their substance use and with making a commitment to change. As we will discuss in greater detail in the chapter on individual treatment (Chapter 5), providing feedback is a powerful tool for intervening with individuals in these two stages of change. In a similar manner, information gathered using these approaches can be used as well with individuals in the preparation stage, where the person is engaged and committed to the change process and on the verge of taking action. Here assessment data can be used for consolidating and building upon that commitment to the change process and in the development of a particular plan of action for that individual.

ASSESSMENTS WITH PARTICULAR RELEVANCE TO CLIENTS IN THE ACTION AND MAINTENANCE STAGES

The tasks of treatment differ as a function of the person's stage of change, as we will describe in upcoming chapters (such as Chapter 5 on individual treatment and Chapter 6 on group treatment). Similarly, the focus of assessment often will vary as a function of the stage of change. Information gathered using the previously presented measures can be used by the therapist and client to generate hypotheses or deductions about the client's substance use and factors associated with its maintenance. The evaluation of such hypotheses is referred to as specialized assessment, which is particularly relevant to individuals in the action and maintenance stages of change. The results of these specialized assessments, each conducted to test a unique hypothesis about a person's alcohol and drug use behavior, are used to develop more refined treatment interventions for a given individual. Accordingly, this section has three major parts. First, we discuss how the assessment measures applied in the context of clients in the precontemplation, contemplation, and preparation stages of change can be used in the specialized assessment of clients who progress into the action and maintenance stages. Second, we introduce and discuss several measures directly relevant to the action and maintenance stages of change. Finally, we discuss considerations in the assessment of relapse risk and self-efficacy.

Specialized Assessment

Several examples will help to clarify the use of this more specialized level of assessment. The first would most likely occur while a person is in treatment and in the action stage of change. Suppose that the Comprehensive Drinker Profile (CDP) was administered to the person as part of the formal intake assessment. Section "C" of the CDP is called "Motivational Information" and concerns reasons for drinking and the effects a person experiences when he or she drinks alcohol. Two items in Section C consist of open-ended questions, respectively, about thoughts or feelings that tend to trigger a desire to drink and situations or a set of events that might result in the person's drinking. Once completed, these two items and the remaining wide-ranging items of the CDP are typical of assessments conducted in the precontemplation, contemplation, and preparation stages; however, psychological and situational triggers to drink can be evaluated in considerably more detail in assessments associated with the action and maintenance stages. One possibility for such a specialized assessment is to ask the individual to complete the Inventory of Drinking Situations (IDS; Annis, Graham, & Davis, 1987), which is described in greater detail later in this chapter. The IDS is a questionnaire that is designed to measure "high risk" situations or triggers for heavy drinking and provides a risk profile of eight factors: unpleasant emotions, physical discomfort, pleasant emotions, testing personal control, urges and temptations to drink, conflict with others, social pressure to drink, and pleasant times with others. If there is consistency between the CDP trigger responses and the IDS, these data could be made the basis of a specialized coping skills training intervention.

We can readily offer a second example of specialized assessment that would be most useful with a person in the action stage of change. As part of a structured diagnostic interview, the mental status exam may suggest that a polysubstance abuser who has been adequately detoxified has short-term memory impairment but no deficits in longer-term memory or in other areas of cognitive functioning. Further testing of this possibility would be critical, as the presence of short-term memory deficits could have considerable influence on how a treatment is administered or affect the content of treatment. A specialized assessment, therefore, would be indicated. In this case, it would make sense to administer the person the Wechsler Memory Scale—Revised, which would result in data on different types (short-term, long-term, verbal, and visual are examples) of memory function. In addition, administration of the Wechsler Intelligence Scale for Adults—Revised (WAIS-R) would enable an extensive evaluation of general intelligence or cognitive functioning. When time restraints exist, the briefer Shipley Institute of Living Scale could be used as a measure of general intelligence.

Another example of specialized assessment is especially applicable to the maintenance stage. In this case, a person completes an inpatient alcohol and drug treatment program. Part of that program involves participation in a social skills group. Systematic behavioral observation of the individual in that group, as well as his or her performance on the Situational Competency Test (a behavioral test of responses in situations that may be high risk for drinking), suggests difficulties in resisting friends' pressure to drink or use drugs but strengths in expressing positive and negative feelings. On these bases, the individual's therapist might well predict that potential relapse situations for the person will center on those in which there might be considerable peer-group pressure to use substances, such as at parties. Therefore, these predispositions would be important to know at the beginning of the maintenance (of sobriety) stage of change and in developing an individual's "aftercare" or discharge plans. One way to proceed with this evaluation would be to ask the person to complete the Situational Confidence Questionnaire (SCQ; Annis & Graham, 1988; also described further later in this chapter). The SCQ is a counterpart to the IDS in that it asks the respondent to indicate how likely he or she will be able to cope with a variety of situations without drinking (a version for other drugs also has been developed). The items on the SCQ generally parallel those on the IDS, and the SCQ yields a profile on the same eight dimensions used in the IDS. Wherever the individual shows less confidence or "self-efficacy" (Bandura, 1977) to cope with different situations without using alcohol or drugs is where relapse theoretically is most probable.

Collecting quantifiable information on a person's functioning greatly helps the effort to evaluate the progress and outcome of treatment through the measurement of change. Therefore, one hypothesis to be tested in specialized assessment is whether treatment is having a given effect(s) in a given area(s) of functioning. Such treatment outcome assessment often is a part of "Total Quality Improvement" evaluations that are expected in clinical settings.

Measures Pertinent to the Action and Maintenance Stages

There are several measures with particular relevance to working with clients in the action and maintenance stages. Two of these measures, the Inventory of Drinking Situations and the Situational Confidence Questionnaire (just alluded to in the context of specialized assessment) are probably the most widely used methods for assessing drinking and drug use and self-efficacy associated with them. In this chapter we will describe them, as well as the Alcohol Abstinence Self-Efficacy Scale, which was developed to assess an individual's efficacy or confidence in abstaining from alcohol in a variety of situations. This measure, which taps both temptations to drink and confidence in abstaining, was found to be a strong predictor of posttreatment drinking behavior among alcoholics (Project MATCH Research Group, 1997b). Taken together, these measures have significant potential use for providing information relevant to treatment planning and the maintenance of treatment gains.

Inventory of Drinking Situations

The original Inventory of Drinking Situations (IDS; Annis, 1982a; Annis et al., 1987) consisted of 100 items designed to assess situations in which the client drank heavily over the past year. A 42-item version also is available (Isenhart, 1991, 1993). Clients are instructed to rate their frequency of "heavy drinking" in each of 100 situations during the past year on a 4-point rating scale (from never to almost always). Eight general categories of drinking situations, based on Marlatt's classification system (Marlatt & Gordon, 1980, 1985), are addressed: unpleasant emotions (e.g., "When I was angry at the way things had turned out"), physical discomfort (e.g., "When I had trouble sleeping"), pleasant emotions (e.g., "When I felt confident and relaxed"), testing personal control (e.g., "When I wondered about my self-control over alcohol and felt like having a drink to try it out"), urges and temptations to drink (e.g., "When I remembered how good it tasted"), conflict with others (e.g., "When other people interfered with my plans"), social pressure to drink (e.g., "When I met a friend and he/she suggested that we have a drink together"), and pleasant times with others (e.g., "When I was relaxed with a good friend and wanted to have a good time").

Clients define heavy drinking in terms of their own consumption pattern and their perception of what constitutes heavy for them. Sobell and Sobell (1993) suggested that clinicians ask clients at the start of the questionnaire to note the number of standard drinks that they consider heavy drinking to provide a reference point for their responses.

A client's "problem index" score, ranging from 1 to 100, can be calculated for each of the eight categories of drinking situations. Plotting the eight problem index scores produces a client profile that shows the areas of greatest risk for heavy drinking and helps target and guide interventions. Those profiles that evidence variability across situations, or differentiated profiles, are more helpful in the identification of specific intervention targets than are generalized or flat profiles with little variation across situations. Clients with differentiated profiles may also have better outcomes in relapse prevention treatment than those with generalized profiles (Annis & Davis, 1991).

Studies of the psychometric properties of the IDS-100 and its 42-item version suggest adequate levels of reliability (Cannon, Leeka, Patterson, & Baker, 1990; Isenhart, 1991, 1993). However, factor analyses at the item level failed to support the presence of the eight rationally derived Marlatt drinking relapse categories. On the original 100-item IDS, Cannon and associates (1990) found three primary factors representing categories of situations in which alcoholics are likely to drink: negative affective states, positive affective states combined with social cues to drink, and attempts to test one's ability to control one's drinking. Isenhart (1991) found five factors, having some conceptual overlap with those obtained by Cannon: negative emotions, social pressure, testing personal control, physical distress, and positive emotions. An item-level principal components analysis replicated this factor structure with the 42-item version, although a second-order principal components analysis at the scale level suggested a single, unitary factor solution (Isenhart, 1993).

The level of specificity in the drinking categories used will vary based on clinical needs. However, Annis and colleagues recommend using the full IDS-100 and the eight relapse risk categories of the original scale for maximal utility in treatment planning and intervention targeting (Annis et al., 1987).

Inventory of Drug-Taking Situations

The Inventory of Drug-Taking Situations (IDTS; Annis & Martin, 1993a) is a 50-item questionnaire whose structure is similar to the IDS. Respondents are instructed to complete the IDTS for their self-identified drug of choice. As with the IDS, the eight subscores derived can be used to identify a drug-taking risk profile for the client.

Situational Confidence Questionnaire

As we noted earlier, the Situational Confidence Questionnaire (SCQ; Annis, 1982b, 1987; Annis & Graham, 1988) is a counterpart to the IDS. The original SCQ consisted of 100 items (now there also are 42- and 39-

item versions of the test) that were created to measure an individual's self-efficacy in coping with different situations without drinking heavily. While the IDS attempts to determine the relative cue strength for drinking in each situation, the SCQ attempts to determine individuals' current level of confidence in their ability to encounter each of these situations without drinking heavily.

Clients are asked to imagine themselves in the same set of drinking situations as presented in the IDS and to rate, on a scale ranging from "not at all confident" to "very confident," how they feel about resisting the urge to drink heavily in that situation. As with the IDS, it appears that fewer than eight meaningful categories of drinking situations are assessed by the SCQ, based on the results of factor analysis. Sandahl, Linberg, and Ronnberg (1990), for instance, found four factors at the item level that parallel those on the IDS: unpleasant emotions, social pressure, testing personal control, and positive emotions.

A client's responses on the SCQ can be used to monitor the development of the client's self-efficacy in relation to coping with specific drinking situations (identified and prioritized by use of the IDS) over the course of treatment or with increasing sobriety. Self-efficacy would be expected to increase across treatment; this appears to be the case (e.g., Burling, Reilly, Molzen, & Ziff, 1989; P. J. Miller, Ross, Emmerson, & Todt, 1989; Rychtarik, Prue, Rapp, & King, 1992; Sitharthan & Kavanagh, 1991). Burling et al. (1989), for example, found that self-efficacy increased during the course of inpatient treatment and was higher for those individuals who were abstainers at a 6-month follow-up than for those who had relapsed.

Presumably, a relative increase in efficacy would occur in those situations that were the focus of intervention (Annis & Davis, 1988). The assumption that higher levels of self-efficacy would be associated with lower levels of relapse or posttreatment drinking has also been supported (e.g., Rychtarik et al., 1992; Sitharthan & Kavanagh, 1991; Solomon & Annis, 1990), although this has not been a universal result (e.g., Mayer & Koeningsmark, 1991). Nevertheless, profiles for the SCQ (and also for the IDS) may be valuable aids in treatment planning and evaluation (Cunningham, Sobell, Sobell, Gavin, & Annis, 1995).

Drug-Taking Confidence Questionnaire

The Drug-Taking Confidence Questionnaire (DTCQ; Annis & Martin, 1993b) is a 50-item measure whose dimensions correspond to the IDTS.

Respondents are asked to rate their degree of confidence in being able to handle situations without using drugs.

Alcohol Abstinence Self-Efficacy Scale

DiClemente, Carbonari, Montgomery, and Hughes (1994) noted that the SCQ may not be an appropriate measure to assess self-efficacy in an abstinence-oriented treatment program. The SCQ focuses on the individual's ability to resist the urge to drink heavily, not necessarily to refrain from drinking completely. They suggest that the goals of treatment (e.g., abstinence or harm reduction) should correspond to the type of efficacy being assessed. As such, they express some concern that efficacy in avoiding drinking heavily as manifested on the SCQ may miss some important aspects of efficacy in remaining abstinent.

To this end, DiClemente, Gordon, and Gibertini (1983) and DiClemente et al. (1994) developed a measure that focuses on the individual's efficacy or confidence in abstaining from alcohol across a range of situations derived from Marlatt's eight primary relapse categories and surveys of drinkers in treatment. The original scale, the Alcohol Abstinence Self-Efficacy Scale (AASE), consists of 49 items. Each item is rated on two separate 5-point scales (from not at all to extremely) to reflect both the temptation to drink and the confidence in abstaining in each situation.

The AASE has been used in conjunction with evaluation of treatment for alcohol-dependent individuals in several studies. Ito, Donovan, and Hall (1988) found that individuals involved following hospitalization in group-administered, relapse-prevention-focused aftercare showed a significant decrease in their level of temptation and an increased level of self-efficacy over the 8-week course. However, clients involved in an interpersonally based aftercare group therapy program demonstrated no significant changes in either temptation or confidence across the corresponding 8-week treatment phase. DiClemente and Hughes (1990) also found that alcoholics entering outpatient treatment who were discouraged, less motivated, and less ready to engage in behavior change activities demonstrated the highest level of temptation and the lowest level of confidence. Finally, in a national study on alcoholism treatment (Project MATCH Research Group, 1997b), confidence scores from the AASE were prognostic of posttreatment drinking among outpatient clients: higher pretreatment confidence was associated with a greater percentage of days abstinent and fewer drinks per drinking day posttreatment. More intriguing was the finding that temptation relative to confidence (calculated as the temptation score on the AASE minus the confidence score) predicted drinking outcomes among outpatients and also among aftercare clients (those who participated in an aftercare treatment that followed a more intensive inpatient or day hospital treatment). For both populations of clients, the higher the temptation minus confidence score, the fewer the percentage of days abstinent during follow-up and the greater average number of drinks per drinking day (DiClemente, Carbonari, Daniels, et al., 2001).

The scale is composed of four factors. The first is a negative affect factor, which includes intrapersonal (e.g., "When I am feeling depressed") and interpersonal (e.g., "When I feel like blowing up because of frustration") negative affect. Social situations (e.g., "When I am being offered a drink in a social situation") and the use of alcohol to enhance positive states (e.g., "When I am excited or celebrating with others") represent a social/positive emotion, the second factor. The third factor, physical and other concerns, consists of varied items representing physical discomfort or pain (e.g., "When I am experiencing some physical pain or injury"), concerns about others (e.g., "When I am concerned about someone"), and dreams about drinking (e.g., "When I dream about taking a drink"). The final factor, withdrawal and urges, represents withdrawal (e.g., "When I am in agony because of stopping or withdrawing from alcohol use"), craving (e.g., "When I am feeling a physical need or craving for alcohol"), and testing willpower (e.g., "When I want to test my willpower over drinking").

Considerations in the Assessment of Relapse Risk and Self-Efficacy

A number of important caveats have been offered by Sobell and colleagues concerning high-risk drinking and drug use situations (and by extension relapse risk) and self-efficacy. While their comments were directed specifically at the IDS and SCQ, in various ways they are applicable to the evaluation of the other questionnaire measures of situational self-efficacy reviewed above. Sobell et al. (1994) noted that the situations identified by measures such as the IDS as potentially risky have only been associated with heavy drinking; therefore, one cannot presume a causal link between the types of situations endorsed, drinking behavior, and relapse probability. A number of other factors, such as coping skills deficits, may represent a common third factor that moderates this relationship.

Second, while the use of such scales to assess temptation, confidence, and coping can be helpful clinically in the treatment planning process, they only identify generic situations or general problem areas. It is important to explore in more depth the unique and personally relevant high-risk situations or areas in which the client lacks self-confidence in resisting drinking or drug use. One might choose to expand more fully on those situations associated with frequent substance use, high temptation ratings, or low levels of perceived confidence on the structured questionnaires. Sobell et al. (1994) also recommend that clinicians ask clients to describe in detail their three highest-risk situations for substance use over the past year.

The latter recommendation is consistent with the recent development and use of semistructured, individualized approaches to the assessment of self-efficacy. K. J. Miller, McCrady, Abrams, and Labouvie (1994), for example, examined the usefulness of an individualized approach to the assessment of self-efficacy in an outpatient alcohol treatment program. An Individualized Self-Efficacy Survey (ISS) was developed for each client. This survey was derived by (1) administering the Drinking Patterns Questionnaire to identify important problem areas for the individual (e.g., work, children, marital problems) and specific drinking antecedents and (2) constructing a 15-item scale using each drinker's most important drinking cues. The method of having clients choose their own high-risk drinking cues appeared to be clinically useful. Ratings on the ISS reflected changes in perceived efficacy over the course of treatment, and ISS scores at the end of treatment predicted subsequent relapse.

A second example of an individualized approach to assessment is the Substance Abuse Relapse Assessment (SARA) developed by Schonfeld and colleagues (Peters & Schonfeld, 1993; Schonfeld, Peters, & Dolente, 1993; Schonfeld, Rohrer, Dupree, & Thomas, 1989). The SARA is a semistructured interview protocol designed to assist clinical staff in developing relapse prevention goals by identifying high-risk situations and deficits in coping skills. It assesses both alcohol and drug use patterns, antecedents or precipitants of drinking and drug use, and positive and negative consequences of drinking. While the focus of the assessment is on a "typical drinking day" over a 30-day period, the interview could easily be adapted to focus on a single or multiple relapse episodes.

In addition to being asked about the parameters of their use patterns, such as the number of days of use and number of days of intoxication, clients are also asked to classify their use patterns as steady, periodic or binge, weekend, or infrequent. The interview focuses on situations, thoughts, feelings, cues, and urges as related to drinking and/or drug use; each of these is assessed as independent categories that are probed for occasions of drinking or substance use.

To provide additional structure to the assessment of emotions as a possible antecedent of drinking, clients are provided with a list of 28 positive and negative emotions and are asked to choose that feeling most prominent immediately before drinking, to explain what the emotion means to them, and to continue doing this until they have rank ordered the five most notable emotions experienced prior to use. Clients are asked how they dealt with these thoughts and feelings on days that they experienced them but did not drink. They are also asked about their responses to prior "slips."

Information derived from the 45- to 60-minute interview is used by the clinician to complete relapse prevention planning forms that provide an overview of clients' substance abuse behavior chain, the current level of necessary coping skills to avoid relapse, the level of confidence the clients have in their ability to avoid relapse, and a set of goals for relapse prevention interventions targeted on those situations, thoughts, feelings, cues, and urges identified as having a high risk for relapse.

SUMMARY

• Assessment is the collection and use of information to obtain an understanding of an individual for purposes of planning treatment, modifying the treatment plan (as warranted) over time, and evaluating treatment progress and outcome.

• There are now several different methods of measuring stage of change. The methods most commonly reported in current literature are the staging algorithm and the University of Rhode Island Change Assessment (URICA) scale, although a few instruments specific to alcohol and drug use are becoming increasingly popular.

• A variety of measures are being used to identify and specify substance misuse. These assessments can be used to provide feedback to indi-

viduals on their substance use and its consequences (particularly to persons in the precontemplation and contemplation stages of change) and to
identify factors associated with the maintenance of substance misuse.

• Several measures are available for assessing individuals in the action
and maintenance stages of change. Of particular relevance are measures to
identify a client's self-efficacy in dealing with situations associated with
risk for drinking or drug use.

4

TREATMENT PLANNING

The treatment plan, one of the most important components of the treatment process, is based on the information gathered during assessment. Developed in collaboration with the client, the treatment plan is designed to address mutually agreed upon treatment goals. The process of carefully and collaboratively developing the treatment plan cannot be overemphasized. The treatment plan organizes, integrates, and prioritizes the material collected during assessment and serves as the plan of action for pursuing the identified goals of treatment. As such, the plan serves a variety of important purposes, including prioritizing short-term and long-term goals, selecting the optimal interventions for specific goals, identifying barriers to the achievement of goals, and monitoring progress toward goals over time (see Donovan, 1995).

This chapter opens with a description of the treatment plan. Following that is a section on developing treatment goals. An emphasis here is placed on incorporating the collaboration of the client in this process. Then we discuss procedures for matching specific treatment activities to treatment goals, previewing in part some of the treatment techniques and strategies that are described in later chapters. Representative treatment plans are presented, the first dealing with an alcohol-dependent client in the contemplation stage and the second with a cocaine-dependent client in the action stage.

THE TREATMENT PLAN

The treatment plan is essentially the agenda that emerges from the assessment process. It is highlighted by a delineation of treatment goals and a corresponding set of clinical interventions designed to assist in the achievement of these goals. The treatment plan is unique to the individual because the presenting needs of clients vary considerably from person to person, as do their available strengths and resources for effecting change. Not surprisingly, the better and more precise the tailoring of the treatment plan to the client's needs and resources, the better the potential fit and the greater the likelihood of achieving the specified treatment goals.

The therapist and client must develop a list of treatment goals and then prioritize those goals. In many cases the primary goal is a decrease in, or cessation of, substance use. Focusing on this goal may have an impact on other key goals, such as improving a family or employment situation. Secondary goals might include extending one's social support network, returning to school, and so on. Whatever the objectives are, it is important to prioritize them. While one obvious benefit of such prioritizing is that attention is focused on the most pressing problem areas, another advantage is that successes in these primary areas, such as cessation of substance use, often place the client in a much better position to subsequently address secondary goals.

As they identify and prioritize goals, the therapist and client also need to specify which are short-term goals and which are long-term. Although there is no consensus about setting these terms, short-term goals often are identified as those that can be significantly addressed within 6 months (e.g., Lewis, Dana, & Blevins, 1988). Long-term goals are those more likely to be achieved over longer periods, although this would not preclude initial efforts to address such goals in the short term and over time. The distinction between short-term and long-term goals is important to highlight, as clients move through the stages of change at different times and paces.

A number of variables will influence the establishment of short-term and long-term goals. As identified by P. M. Miller and Mastria (1977), one of the key factors is the extent and seriousness of the problem. Any pretreatment evaluation of a substance will include assessment of severity of dependence and need for detoxification or some other form of medical management. By necessity, problems in this domain would require immediate attention.

Goal setting is influenced as well by the nature and extent of the client's motivation to invest in and pursue treatment goals. An assessment of the client's stage of change will yield some insights into his or her extent of readiness to embark on the change process. The client in contemplation will likely be vacillating between the advantages and disadvantages to making changes in his or her life. A client in the action stage will be more ready than one in an earlier stage to start the change process and much less likely to want to devote time and energy to deciding on whether to commit to change.

The determination that a client is in the contemplation or action stage of change does not preclude the full development of the treatment plan, but it has implications for how the treatment goals are established and operationalized. A possible short-term goal for the person in the contemplation stage would be evaluation of the pros and cons of making changes in substance use patterns, using principles of motivational counseling (Miller & Rollnick, 1991) and decisional balance exercises (Janis & Mann, 1977). Short-term goals for the client in the action stage could include, as examples, attendance at self-help groups and problem solving alternatives to substance use, as such clients are going to be more ready to embark on such change efforts.

It is important that whatever goals are identified be achievable, and that procedures be established to allow the client to take small and progressive steps in gradually achieving the goals. There are two reasons for adhering to such a strategy. The first is that complex problems are not generally amenable to easy, one-step solutions, regardless of the person's level of motivation. Rather, breaking down the problem into its subcomponents and successively addressing these is both a more manageable and a more successful approach to the larger problem. Second, developing a step-wise plan for addressing problems sets the stage for the client to experience a series of small but meaningful successes in pursuit of his or her goals. This is particularly important when the client is not fully confident about his or her ability to succeed in the change process. Experiencing some initial successes lessens the likelihood of the discouragements clients often experience when their expectations or goals for treatment are too ambitious. Such discouragements are a major contributor to dropping out of treatment.

P. M. Miller and Mastria (1977) have identified several other factors that can influence the development of short-term and long-term treatment goals. These include the treatment setting, the availability of significant others, and the projected period of treatment involvement. In terms of setting, for example, short-term goals for clients in an inpatient unit will differ in certain ways from those established for outpatient clients. Outpatients have the benefit of trying out treatment strategies in their actual living environments but do not have the benefits of the more protective inpatient unit, which affords more opportunities for regrouping and consolidation. Availability of significant others and their investment in the client can influence the plans for achieving treatment goals. For example, spouses, other family members, and friends may be available to participate in treatment sessions or can be called upon by the client in other ways to support and contribute to his or her efforts to make changes.

Finally, the projected treatment period can markedly influence treatment planning. The treatment plan for a client allocated three months of outpatient treatment will differ from that developed for a client with the opportunity for a lengthier treatment intervention. Insurance policies can determine treatment periods, but clients themselves bring their own expectations about how long treatment should last—and such expectations need to be acknowledged and respected. For the client who expects treatment to be briefer than the therapist thinks advisable, negotiating a treatment plan that incorporates a compromise duration, at the end of which the plan and progress to date would be reviewed, may be possible.

It is important that the client and therapist alike recognize the treatment plan as flexible and changeable. They should view the initial treatment plan, based on the pretreatment assessment and evaluation, as a working blueprint for change, and both should understand and acknowledge that changes can—and likely *will*—be made in it over time. As such, treatment planning actually is a continuous and dynamic component of the treatment process. There are several reasons for this (Sobell et al., 1982). First, there may be some needs or problems that are not apparent during the pretreatment assessment. Second, progress on some treatment goals may need to await progress on other problem areas. In such cases, it may be necessary to rearrange treatment goal priorities. Third, some problems may take longer to address than other problems or than originally anticipated. Revisions of the treatment plan will help the client and therapist keep abreast of relative progress in the pursuit of treatment goals. Finally, it is not unusual for new problems to arise during treatment, problems that may require immediate incorporation into the treatment plan.

While treatment programs often allow some latitude in the format and content of treatment plans, there nevertheless are external influences, such as state and other regulatory and oversight organizations, that have concrete guidelines on what constitutes an acceptable treatment plan. One organization that has widespread influence in this regard is the Joint Commission on Accreditation of Healthcare Organizations (JCAHO). Their manuals outline the requirements of an acceptable treatment plan, the highlights of which are listed in Table 4.1.

One point listed in Table 4.1 that we have not yet discussed is the incorporation, as warranted, of interdisciplinary inputs. For example, each substance-abusing client should receive a physical exam and workup. In this context, the potential use of pharmacotherapy can be evaluated. Disulfiram and naltrexone have been used with some benefits among alcoholics, and methadone and naltrexone have potential benefits in the treatment of opioid dependence. (The individual and combined uses of psychotherapy and pharmacotherapy are discussed in greater detail by Carroll, 1996a.)

TABLE 4.1. Common Features of an Individualized Treatment Plan

Developed as a result of a comprehensive assessment and modified over time as warranted.

Reflects participation from appropriate disciplines (e.g., medicine, psychiatry, psychology, social work, vocational rehabilitation) as warranted.

Reflects the client's presenting needs and specifies the person's strengths and limitations.

Consists of specific goals that pertain to the attainment, maintenance, and/or reestablishment of physical and emotional health.

Identifies specific objectives that relate directly to the treatment goals.

Identifies the services and/or settings necessary for meeting the client's needs and goals.

Specifies the frequency of treatment contacts.

Includes provisions for periodic (and at other times, as indicated by changes in the client's life-functioning) reevaluations and revisions, as warranted, of the treatment plan.

Identifies specific criteria for determining whether goals have been achieved and for terminating treatment.

Note. Data from Joint Commission on Accreditation of Healthcare Organizations (1994, pp. 22–23).

DEVELOPING INDIVIDUALIZED TREATMENT GOALS

While the formulation of treatment goals on the surface may appear to be a fairly mechanical task, in fact it requires a dynamic and collaborative interplay between the client and therapist on the identification of needs. Many of the assessment tools we identified in Chapter 3 are particularly relevant to this process.

In almost all cases, current substance use and its consequences are a primary concern. Treatment goals concerning substance abuse, as with all other treatment objectives, need to be clearly identified, since the absence of explicit goals would make it difficult for the therapist and especially the client to evaluate progress and success (Berg & Miller, 1992). Wherever possible, express treatment goals positively. As noted by Sobell et al. (1982), goals stated positively allow greater possibilities for producing behavior change. The positively stated goal of "achieve and maintain progressively longer periods of abstinence from crack" may hold more promise than the alternative goal of "stop getting high." Relatedly, it is often more effective to state goals in terms of increasing desired behaviors rather than focusing on decreasing unwanted behaviors.

An individual's substance abuse is almost always associated with various forms of life dysfunction, whether in the marital, family, vocational, health, or legal domains. Accordingly, treatment planning needs to give cognizance to all these areas, even though in many cases the initiation of abstinence or significant reductions in substance use will alleviate at least some of the more acute problems. In addition, substance use is often associated with other comorbid psychiatric disturbances, such as depression or anxiety (e.g., Regier et al., 1990; Ross, Glaser, & Germanson, 1988), and these issues require corresponding attention.

Regardless of the nature of the particular problem area, the same essential issues need to be kept in mind in developing the respective treatment goals. A listing of the key qualities of well-formed treatment goals, many of which have already been mentioned, is provided in Table 4.2.

Wherever possible, the goals of the treatment plan should reflect the client's goals, not the therapist's. Doing so affords the client a greater sense of ownership and potential responsibility for whatever treatment objectives emerge from the treatment planning process. Furthermore, clients more often than not decide for themselves, either before or after the initiation of treatment, the goals they consider primary. Clients by and large will decide and act upon their own substance abuse goals even if they are

**TABLE 4.2. Some Qualities of
Well-Formed Treatment Goals**

Salient and meaningful to the client

Incremental and thus more manageable

Concrete, specific, and behavior focused

Focused on increasing desired behaviors

Include progressive steps for achieving goals

Realistic and achievable

Perceived as requiring work and effort

Appropriate for the projected treatment period

Note. Adapted in part from Berg and Miller (1992).

at variance with the treatment program goals (e.g., Sanchez-Craig, Annis, Bornet, & MacDonald, 1984; Miller, Leckman, Delaney, & Tinkcom, 1992; Nordstrom & Berglund, 1987). Several studies have shown that better treatment outcomes are associated with treatment goals being consistent with the client's goal preference (Booth, Dale, & Ansari, 1984; Orford & Keddie, 1986).

Throughout the assessment and treatment planning process—indeed, from the point of initial contact—the therapist needs to engender a productive working alliance with the client and enhance the client's motivation to change. While some clients enter the treatment process highly motivated and ready for taking action, most present with reservations. Such clients are typically in the contemplation phase, and with these clients in particular therapists should key on strategies for increasing motivation to change and for keeping clients engaged in the processes surrounding development and implementation of the treatment plan.

One useful approach to increasing the likelihood of sustained treatment involvement is motivational enhancement. When used in the early stages of treatment, motivation-enhancing techniques reduce premature attrition and help to engender greater treatment participation. We previewed such interventions in Chapter 2 in the context of reconceptualizing denial and resistance. Here we will describe in greater detail some techniques for increasing motivation to change.

Miller and Sanchez (1994) have identified some factors that appear to increase clients' motivation to change. The acronym FRAMES has been used to summarize these strategies, which include the following:

Feedback of information from assessment, emphasis on personal *Responsibility* for change, *Advice* to change, providing a *Menu* of strategies for change, therapist *Empathy*, and facilitation of client *Self-efficacy*. Motivational interviewing (see Miller & Rollnick, 1991; Miller, Zweben, DiClemente, & Rychtarik, 1992) incorporates the FRAMES components with the specific objective of increasing client motivation. In the context of intake and treatment planning sessions, motivational interviewing would entail the therapist's use of specific listening and questioning strategies to assist clients in working through ambivalence about making changes in their substance use behavior.

Given that many clients entering treatment are ambivalent about change, we will describe briefly how principles of motivational interviewing, as summarized in the FRAMES acronym, might be used during the intake and treatment planning sessions to reduce or prevent resistance, to engage the client in the treatment endeavor, and to increase cooperation with the treatment process. In almost all initial sessions, the therapist naturally would elicit from the client a description, in the client's own words, of the presenting problem and the factors contributing to his or her seeking treatment at this time. Using principles of motivational interviewing, the therapist would convey *empathy* through use of reflective listening techniques. At whatever point the therapist has accumulated sufficient information, the therapist would provide a summary of the concerns voiced by the client and *feedback* of indications garnered through the assessment process. This feedback could include topics such as the frequency, intensity, and duration of substance use; problems directly and indirectly associated with such use; other areas of functioning, such as mood; comparisons of indications from the assessment to norms from the general population and/or from treatment-seeking samples; and risk factors, such as family history or environmental factors, that might suggest an increased susceptibility to continued or worsening difficulties. The emphasis in these interactions should be on describing the client's functioning in terms that are meaningful to the client, as opposed to presenting a formal diagnosis. Often it is useful to provide the client with a written summary of the feedback to review later.

With the foregoing as foundation, the therapist is now in a position to help the client gauge for himself or herself the relative strength and importance of the costs and benefits of change. In doing so, the therapist would be attempting to move the client toward a greater commitment to change. The therapist makes clear to the client that the *responsibility* for deciding what, if anything, to do about his or her substance use is the client's. At the same time, the therapist provides clear *advice* to change. As part of the process of identifying strategies for addressing treatment goals, the therapist can provide a *menu* of options for change, ideally based on clinical research regarding effective treatments for substance misuse. Finally, the therapist engenders client *self-efficacy* by stressing that treatment is likely to be successful if the client is committed to making a change.

Throughout the intake and treatment planning sessions, the therapist can utilize a variety of strategies to move the client toward a determination that change is necessary, desirable, and achievable. These techniques, taken from Miller, Zweben, et al. (1992), include the following:

- *Elicit self-motivational statements.* Self-motivational statements are those that reflect the client's openness to feedback on his or her substance use, an acknowledgment of problems associated to date with such use, and expressions of the need or willingness to make change. One of the most fruitful ways of eliciting such statements entails the use of open-ended questions.

- *Listen with empathy.* Sometimes called reflection, or active listening, this technique entails listening carefully to statements made by the client and then reflecting them back on the client. Such responses encourage the client to continue talking and are not likely to elicit resistance, both important advantages in early treatment sessions. Importantly, listening with empathy demonstrates the therapist's respect for and interest in the client, which contributes in turn to the development of a productive therapeutic alliance.

- *Ask open-ended questions.* Asking the client about his or her feelings, concerns, and plan is more productive than telling the client how he or she should feel or what he or she needs to do.

- *Affirm the client.* Affirming and complimenting the client in a way that acknowledges his or her serious consideration of and steps toward change can improve the treatment process.

- *Handle resistance.* One productive strategy for dealing with client resistance is to deflect it by simply reflecting the client's feelings or by shifting focus away from the problematic issue, rather than debating with or confronting the client.

- *Reframe.* The therapist can restate client perceptions in a form more likely to be conducive to and supportive of making change. In this fashion, new meanings and perspectives are provided to the client.

- *Summarize.* The therapist can consolidate the material presented by the client over the course of the session in a positive and realistic way. Summaries that reflect and repeat self-motivational statements made by the client are particularly helpful.

These clinical strategies are described in much greater detail elsewhere by Miller and his colleagues (W. R. Miller, 1995; Miller & Rollnick, 1991; Miller, Zweben, et al., 1992; Rollnick, Mason, & Butler, 1999). The use of these techniques, taken together, have great potential for engaging the client in a productive and well-planned treatment process.

APPLYING SPECIFIC TREATMENT ACTIVITIES TO TREATMENT GOALS

Once treatment goals have been identified, it becomes necessary to match them with treatment activities designed to accomplish them. Most treatment objectives are multifaceted, and even in their simplest forms there will be several treatment options potentially available for application. Accordingly, the therapist needs to evaluate treatment options in relation to the various treatment goals and determine which strategies to select, keeping in mind the client's unique strengths and resources. In addition, the client's current readiness to change will influence the nature of treatment options selected. For example, the use of action-focused techniques for abstaining from substance use may not be productive in the early stages of treatment with an individual who is only contemplating such change. Similarly, evaluating the pros and cons of making behavior change will not be particularly timely with the client who is already in the action stage of change.

While the fit between the individual's needs and capabilities and the treatment strategies is instrumental in fostering early progress in treatment, the treatment activities should not be viewed as etched in stone. Instead, the treatment activities associated with a particular goal can be modified as a function of progress toward that goal. In addition, it sometimes is necessary to utilize other treatment strategies if the client's circumstances change, such as when the severity of substance use increases beyond that presented at treatment entry. Flexibility in applying specific treatment activities is central to an individualized approach to a client's needs.

The range of treatment strategies potentially available for use in working with substance-abusing clients is wide, and in subsequent chapters we will discuss a variety of treatment activities, including strategies for use in individual treatment and group treatment formats. The case studies that follow pick up on those we presented in Chapter 2 and illustrate the development and implementation of individualized treatment plans.

REPRESENTATIVE TREATMENT PLANS

Case Example 1: Treatment Plan for an Alcohol-Dependent Client in the Contemplation Stage

As we discussed in Chapter 2, Maureen J is a 46-year-old divorced woman presenting at a community mental health center because she is drinking more than she would like and is thinking about quitting. Almost all of her drinking occurs with friends and other patrons in a local tavern that is close to where she works and lives. On Mondays she generally is abstinent. On Tuesdays, Wednesdays, and Thursdays she typically consumes three to five bottles of beer each day. On weekends she drinks more heavily, usually 10 to 12 beers a day. She acknowledges a variety of negative consequences of past drinking and is concerned about more potential consequences (especially in the context of driving after drinking at the tavern). Such consequences, taken together, have put her in a position of thinking more about her alcohol use and the possibility of quitting. This is countered, in her mind, by the fact she really has not been "burned" by her drinking and by her belief that important relationships with her friends will be negatively affected if she is not drinking and thus is not one of the gang. As such, she is unclear as to what she needs to do and about what she wants to do about her drinking. For that reason, she contacted the clinic.

Maureen and her counselor discussed her goals and developed the following treatment plan based on them.

Treatment Plan

Long-term goals

1. Sustained abstinence from alcohol as well as any other addictive substances
2. Acquisition and maintenance of meaningful and fulfilling social relationships

3. Acquisition and use of skills to recognize and deal with high-risk situations for re-lapse

Short-term objectives

Goal	Intervention
1. Identification of negative consequences of drinking	Conduct comprehensive alcohol and drug use history, via interview and questionnaire measures, to identify drinking consequences in life-functioning domains (e.g., work, family, social, physical, legal). Refer for physical examination and laboratory workup.
2. Evaluation of pros and cons of drinking	Provide objective feedback on drinking behaviors and pattern (especially since client evaluates drinking in context of how friends drink). Conduct decisional balance exercise to identify and weigh advantages of quitting drinking relative to disadvantages of quitting. Use motivational procedures specifically in this regard to maximize prospects for moving client beyond contemplation.
3. Implement plans to not drive after drinking and to reduce other alcohol-related risks	Develop plans to avoid driving after drinking, such as using a taxi. Identify and address other areas of potential risk similarly, as indicated.
4. Evaluate alternative environments for social ties	Investigate alternative environments for socializing, such as meeting friends in alcohol-free contexts. Explore avenues for meeting new friends and evaluate and address conversational skills, etc., as warranted.
5. Establish short-term abstinence	Initiate as warranted (i.e., as a function of client consent) an initial 30-day period of abstinence. Monitor cravings for alcohol and situational challenges to abstinence. Discuss techniques and strategies to deal with drinking situations (e.g., drink refusal training). Discuss alternatives to drinking (e.g., meeting friends in nondrinking situations).

Attend self-help groups such as Alcoholics Anonymous during this period and evaluate with client benefits experienced.

Discuss over time advantages and disadvantages of not drinking in context of decisional balance.

6. Further engage client in therapeutic endeavor	Provide support and encouragement for collaborative change effort.
	Foster confidence and efficacy on part of client by focusing on initially small steps toward change, thus providing early success experiences.

Comments

Treatment will entail weekly sessions for the first 6 months, with additional sessions during this period scheduled as warranted. Sessions for following 6 months will be tapered according to client status and needs. Treatment plan will be reviewed and updated accordingly at least every 3 months.

Case Example 2: Treatment Plan for a Cocaine-Dependent Client in the Action Stage

As described in Chapter 2, Paul J is a 34-year-old single man who reported using multiple substances in various combinations since junior high school. During the past 6 years his drug use entailed almost daily use of marijuana and alcohol and use of cocaine approximately four times a week. He noted that he occasionally would also use stimulants but that such use was infrequent (maybe once a month, he estimated). His drug use occurred with various combinations of acquaintances from a core group of around 15 persons. That is, he was part of a group of around 15 people who in different combinations would get together. Paul did not spend much time with these individuals beyond these specific drug use contexts.

Paul's drug use over the past decade had precluded the development of significant or long-term relationships with women (and often with friends more generally) and created difficulties maintaining gainful employment. In fact, he had spent most of the past 10 years either underemployed, on unemployment benefits, or on welfare support. The status that bothered him most was underemployment because he felt he was capable of more challenging positions. He noted, with some pride, that his drug use had not led to problems in his physical health (at least, as far as he was aware), accidents, or arrests. It was the absence of problems in these areas that he in the past had used as evidence that he did not have a problem with drug use.

At intake, Paul reported that he wanted to be abstinent from all substance use, including alcohol, and immediately wanted to start taking the steps necessary to achieve this goal. Although asserting the same in the past, he reported it was different this time because he "really" had decided to make changes. As proof of this commitment, he noted that he had not used any alcohol or drugs during the past 5 days, had attended his intake session, had begun to attend self-help group meetings, and had begun to spend time with acquaintances who did not use drugs.

Paul discussed his specific goals with his counselor, and together they drafted a treatment plan.

Treatment Plan

Long-term goals

1. Establish and maintain total abstinence from all addictive substances
2. Acquisition and maintenance of meaningful and fulfilling social relationships
3. Acquisition and use of skills to recognize and deal with high-risk situations for relapse
4. Stable employment consistent with his capabilities

Short-term objectives

Goal	Intervention
1. Identification of negative consequences of drug use	Conduct comprehensive drug use history, via interview and questionnaire measures, to identify drug use consequences in life-functioning domains (e.g., work, family, social, physical, legal). Refer for physical examination and laboratory workup.
2. Establish and maintain abstinence	Contract for continuation of the 5-day abstinent period client brought to intake. Monitor signs of withdrawal. Monitor cravings for drugs.

Monitor contacts with drug-using friends.

Apply strategies to deal with cravings (e.g., relaxation training, alternative activities) and invitations to use (e.g., refusal skills, assertiveness).

Identify alternatives to drug use (e.g., preplanning evening activities with family or non-drug-using friends) to preclude getting together with drug-using friends.

Attend self-help groups, such as Narcotics Anonymous or Cocaine Anonymous, at least 3 times per week.

3. Initiate vocational planning

Referral for vocational counseling to identify areas of strength.

Review classified advertisements and other outlets to identify employment opportunities.

Practice interviewing skills, including explanation for sporadic work history to date.

4. Expand scope of social contacts

Identify non-drug-using friends.

Identify and attend functions not associated with drug use (e.g., seminars, classes).

Comments

Treatment will entail biweekly sessions for the first 3 months, with additional sessions added as needed. These sessions will focus primarily on short-term objectives 1 and 2. Assuming progress on objectives 1 and 2, attention will shift to objectives 3 and 4. Weekly sessions are planned for months 3–6; scheduling of subsequent sessions will be evaluated at that point in time. Treatment plan will be reviewed and updated accordingly at least every 3 months.

APPRECIATING THE DIVERSITY OF CLIENTS

The development of an individualized treatment plan requires a sensitivity to and appreciation of the wide diversity represented by the clients with whom we work. The factor most often taken into account is ethnic and racial background. However, as noted by Miller (1999), clients differ as well along the important dimensions of gender, age, education, socioeconomic status, sexual orientation, and psychological health. Accordingly, clinicians will need to be sensitive to these dimensions of diversity in their evaluation of assessment data, in the development of treatment goals, and in the application of interventions focused on behavior change.

SUMMARY

• The treatment plan, developed in collaboration with the client, is intended to address treatment goals. It organizes, integrates, and prioritizes the information gathered during the assessment process.

• The plan is highlighted by a delineation of treatment goals and a corresponding set of clinical interventions.

• Treatment objectives typically are prioritized and divided as well into short-term and long-term goals.

• The establishment of short-term and long-term goals is influenced by a variety of factors, including extent and seriousness of the substance use problem, client motivational readiness to change, the availability of significant others, and the projected period of treatment involvement.

• Treatment plans should be viewed as flexible and changeable.

• Qualities of well-formed treatment goals include being salient and meaningful to the client, manageable, specific, and appropriate for the projected treatment period.

• In developing the treatment plan, the therapist needs to attend as well to engendering a productive working alliance with the client and enhancing the client's motivation to change.

• Treatment plans need to reflect an appreciation of client diversity.

5

INDIVIDUAL TREATMENT

Individual treatment is uniquely suited to the concepts of the stages of change model. Moving forward through the stages of change requires individuals to resolve different types of problems and to address the tasks and challenges presented by each of the stages (DiClemente, Carbonari, & Velasquez, 1992). What the person in precontemplation needs to do to move out of the precontemplation stage is much different from what he or she will need to do when he or she arrives at the action stage. When an individual will move from contemplation and decide to create a plan of action depends on a variety of unique circumstances and on individual effort. Moreover, each action plan depends on the skills and circumstances of the individual substance abuser. The path to sobriety for each individual will differ as he or she meets the various challenges along the way. Individual treatment ideally is designed to track and assist each client in moving forward in the process of change. The individual therapist is in a position to provide the assistance, resources, and support the client needs to move effectively and efficiently through the various stages of change toward recovery.

The first task of a therapist meeting the client in treatment is to assess where the individual stands in the process of changing his or her substance abuse behaviors. In the assessment chapter, we outlined and discussed the various ways that stage of change and related client change variables can be evaluated on entry to treatment. After the therapist has a good sense of what stage the individual is in, then individualized interventions can proceed. Since stage of change is conceptualized as a state and not a trait, it is productive to continue checking where the individual is located in the process of change. Substance abusers can move around in the stages from day to day and week to week, and even during a session. Stage status is a dynamic—not static—characteristic of the client. Although some individuals can stay in the same stage for long periods (Carbonari, DiClemente, & Sewell, 1999), the potential for swift movement and sudden shifts in stage status is both understandable and documented (Wholey, 1984). The notion of stage as a state and not a trait implies that it is better to think about clients as being "in precontemplation" rather than "being precontemplators." As we described in the initial chapters, each stage represents a series of tasks that need to be accomplished. Stage-specific tasks offer direction as to the approach to be taken and the strategies to employ, and even the type of interpersonal stance that may best promote change (DiClemente & Prochaska, 1998; Prochaska & Norcross, 1994; DiClemente et al., 1992).

This chapter describes how to evaluate stage status in the course of treatment as well as critical tasks and suggested intervention techniques that could be used at each of the stages of change. Case examples are used to illustrate issues and strategies. Changing substance abuse behavior requires shifts in multiple areas of an individual's functioning and environment (DiClemente, 1999a). For each of the stages we discuss what may need to occur in the functioning and in the environment of a client and highlight some strategies to accomplish these changes or shifts. There are some processes that appear to be critical in making the transition from one stage to the next. We highlight these and offer some strategies for engaging these processes. The list of strategies is never exhaustive, as clinicians search continually for new ways to influence clients or new techniques to promote movement through the stages. The search for new and unique ways to influence the process of change represents one of the most creative and dynamic aspects of individual therapy.

ASSESSING THE STAGES OF CHANGE
IN A CLINICAL SETTING

As identified in Chapter 3, a variety of strategies have been developed to assess where individuals stand in the process of changing their substance use (DiClemente & Hughes, 1990; Belding, Iguchi, Lamb, Lakin, & Terry, 1995; Carney & Kivlahan, 1995; Isenhart, 1994). Many of these assessment techniques are readily adaptable for ongoing use throughout the course of treatment. This is important to emphasize, as individuals can move from one stage to the next and even slip back to an earlier stage from week to week, or even day to day. Consequently, ongoing clinical assessment is imperative. Even with an assignment to stage based on a measure administered at intake, the clinician must always check on that status to be aware of the current stage of change. Stage status cannot be captured for the duration of treatment with a single measure taken at intake. Instead, it is important to view stage status as we do drinking or drug use status. For example, when clinicians want to be sure that a client is not using drugs, they can collect a urine sample each time the client comes in for assessment or treatment. The assumption is that drug use status can change at any point from one visit to the next. With stage of change, similarly, the client can shift from one time point to the next. Accordingly, clinicians need to be in a position to assess the client's stage of change frequently, ideally in a manner that is not too obtrusive or burdensome. A sensitive assessment and discussion of stage status at the beginning of each session is an easy and efficient way to track stage for a particular client.

The challenge for the clinician doing a stage status assessment by interview is to gain an accurate understanding of client attitudes and behavior. Judgments about any particular client at any specific time can be erroneous. Clients and therapists often see things differently. In a recent study of the therapeutic alliance, therapists had rather low levels of agreement with their clients in responses to questions about important dimensions of the therapy relationship (Connors, Carroll, DiClemente, Longabaugh, & Donovan, 1997; Connors et al., 2000). In settings in which clients feel that they must give "right" answers or tell you what you want to hear, clients are less likely to make or share accurate self-appraisals. Clinical judgments based on quick impressions, biased assumptions, or poor listening can contribute to inaccurate evaluations of clients. To assess stage of change accurately, the therapist needs to allow the client to be open and listen to what the client is thinking and doing with respect to the problem. The following vignettes represent a second session with two different clients.

Armand arrived about 5 minutes late for his therapy session, complaining about the traffic. He immediately began talking about his wife,

Anne, and her hypercritical way of managing the children. He described in detail several incidents that illustrated his concerns, recounting several confrontations between his wife and their 10-year-old daughter, Amanda. One of these incidents occurred the morning of the session and so was fresh in Armand's mind. When the discussion finally got back to talking about his drinking problem, Armand said that he had been "working on it." Contrary to his usual pattern, he declined an invitation to go out with his business associates on Friday evening. He was proud of this and felt that it proved that he had some control over his drinking. However, he had been drinking at home throughout the weekend. As he discussed his drinking, he mentioned that not drinking would present a real dilemma for him since he would have to change his business lifestyle. In addition, he acknowledged he would need to find other ways to manage his anger at Anne for her rigidity. Drinking helped him escape from his frustration at home.

Bill arrived at his session on time and was accompanied by his wife Barbara. At the beginning of the session he asked if Barbara could join in the session since she was concerned about the treatment and wanted to know more about his problem. He did drink a substantial amount of alcohol over the weekend and had been discussing the possibility of his being an "alcoholic" with Barbara. She was very disturbed by this revelation and the "alcoholic" characterization. Bill now believed he had a serious drinking problem and that it was time to do something. He had been thinking about how to solve the problem when he and his wife had this discussion about abstinence and about being an alcoholic. Barbara was very concerned that their social life would be threatened if he needed to be abstinent.

It is apparent that Bill and Armand are in different places with respect to changing their drinking. Armand does not appear ready to move out of precontemplation, although there are glimmers of insight and contemplation stage activity. The focus on associated problems, such as his wife's child management skills and personal characteristics, provides a related but distinct sidebar and is a sign that he is not ready to focus on his own behavior. It would be a much different situation if he were trying to problem solve the child management issues in order to focus on his drinking. However, without discussing clearly how child management and his drinking were related, Armand is communicating that he is not ready to consider changing his drinking behavior at this time. An unwillingness to focus thought and energy onto consideration of the problem or change is a sign of precontemplation. Armand's acknowledgment that losing his drinking would have some serious other consequences is a beginning consideration but focuses on a reason not to change rather than a reason to change.

Bill, on the other hand, has moved through the contemplation stage and is entering preparation. The tasks that are a main focus of one particular stage often continue to need attention throughout the entire process of change (DiClemente & Prochaska, 1998; Prochaska & DiClemente, 1998). Evaluating the pros and cons, which is a primary task of the contemplation stage, continues into the preparation stage. In fact, Bill's wife Barbara is raising concerns that Bill must now evaluate as potential cons for change. These considerations may encourage him to back off from making a plan and to return to the contemplation stage of change. Bill's acknowledgment that he has a serious problem with drinking and that something must be done is a sign of preparation stage activity. The plan is not yet developed, so there is additional work to be accomplished to move forward into action. However, the tasks of preparation have begun. The challenge is to help him continue his movement forward and to neutralize the concerns of his wife so that they do not interfere with his efforts. There is certainly an indication in his opening remarks that the involvement of his spouse would be an important addition to the treatment endeavor.

As becomes evident from this assessment of stage status, the strategies and topics of intervention are developed as the stage status unfolds. There are several important points to remember about assessing stage status clinically. These elements are part of every good interview and an integral part of motivational interviewing (Miller & Rollnick, 1991).

1. *Listen.* If the therapist begins by talking and asking too many questions, particularly questions that are closed-ended (ones that can be answered with a yes or no) or directive (you are working on your plan, aren't you), it will be difficult to assess stage accurately. The fact that a client drank or used drugs during the past week does not automatically indicate his or her stage. Continuing abstinence is a good sign and often indicative of action or maintenance stage status unless the abstinence represents an imposed or coerced state (stopping drinking or drug use simply to prove that one does not have a problem or to satisfy some external demand). Answers to questions like "Did you drink? Would you like to stop? Can you quit?" do not automatically allow the therapist to

assess stage. Listening to the client's thought process and the content of concerns is the most productive way to observe and assess client status in the process of change (Rollnick et al., 1999).

2. *Ask probing, open-ended questions.* It is most often useful to seek additional information by trying to get the client's perspective and not that of the wife, coworker, or probation officer. Stage assignment must be based on the client's actions, attitudes, and views (DiClemente & Prochaska, 1998). The number of individuals who are nagging him or her or the number of consequences experienced do not measure client commitment to change. In fact, pressure to change can result in two very different responses from the client. Sometimes pressure can provoke thoughtful consideration of the problem and the possibility of change. At other times, pressure or confrontation brings with it feigned compliance and a hardening of resistance to change (Miller, Benefield, & Tonigan, 1993). Only by asking open-ended questions and being open to all the possible responses can a therapist gain access to these reactions.

3. *Check your perceptions.* One of the most useful motivational interviewing strategies for making an accurate assessment of stage status is summarizing (Miller & Rollnick, 1991). This would include periodically checking whether you, the therapist, have it right, asking if the client means this or that, repeating what you heard, and offering a summary in your own words of what you have heard from the client in terms of his or her stage status. These strategies can assist the therapist in understanding client intentions and help ensure what the therapist understands as a pro or con for drinking or drug use really has that same meaning for the client. Again, it is only with accurate information from the client that the therapist can determine where the client is in the process of change.

4. *Review stage status regularly.* If the client is moving forward through the stages, as Bill appears to be, the work the therapist does in the session can help the client to engage in the specific processes of change that produce movement. Reviewing stage status at the end of the session as well as at the beginning is another important strategy. Clients generally make the transitions from one stage to the next on their own during the time between sessions. After the session they have time to reflect and become more engaged in specific process activity. While therapists sometimes may be able to observe clients move forward out of precontemplation and into contemplation or from contemplation to preparation during a session, this is atypical because such transitions often are difficult to capture and occur in the personal space of the client. In either case, it is important

to check regularly on stage status so as to be able to determine when clients are making these transitions from one stage to another. It also is important to remember that regression is almost as likely as progression in the stages, so sensitivity to movement in either direction is warranted. Establishing an understanding of stage status and tracking that status over time is at the heart of matching individual interventions to client stage of change. After a respectful exploration of the client's stage status, the intervention plan can be developed. Of course, that plan would need to be revised as needed based upon the movement or lack of movement through the stages of change.

MEETING THE CLIENT AT EACH STAGE OF CHANGE

Precontemplation Stage

Individual therapy with a client in precontemplation allows the therapist to explore the reasons why this person has come into treatment as well as ways to move him or her from precontemplation. A naive observer might assume that no individuals in a precontemplation stage would come into a treatment program, since only those who want to change would come to treatment. However, reports from clinical studies as well as from clinicians on the front lines indicate that many individuals come to treatment not prepared to change (Simpson & Joe, 1993; Simpson, Joe, Rowan-Szal, & Greener, 1995; Ryan, Plant, & O'Malley, 1995). There are many reasons for seeking treatment that do not include changing substance use behaviors. The most obvious reason is a criminal justice referral to treatment. Judges, probation officers, and lawyers often tell an individual that they must go to treatment to satisfy some legal judgment or to impress the legal system. Individuals in mandated treatment often attend and "cooperate" without any real intention to change their behavior. The personal goal for these individuals is to satisfy the legal system and get out of trouble. For others the rationale is similar but the scenario different. Many are clients who simply want to satisfy a wife or husband who is threatening to leave, parents who have become fed up with the behavior, or employers who want something done to solve problems at work. Another group of individuals in precontemplation may be seeking confirmation that they do *not* have a problem. Finally, some individuals come in to treatment with a goal of changing others and not themselves. There are, of course, many variations on these themes. However, when therapists look closely at their intakes and their caseloads, they often discover a number of the treatment seekers to be in precontemplation for changing their substance use behavior even though they may be cooperating at a superficial level with program requirements (Isenhart, 1994; Donovan, 1999). Many clients openly admit that their primary motivation for seeking treatment is to satisfy an external demand. Motivation for treatment is not the same as motivation for change (DiClemente, 1999b).

Traditional approaches to addressing the precontemplator in treatment have included skepticism, advice, and a healthy dose of confrontation. Advice has often taken the form of labeling ("You are a drug addict" or "You are an alcoholic") and an attempt to convince the client in precontemplation that he or she has a serious problem (Johnson, 1986). This type of advice-giving is likely to benefit only those clients who are in precontemplation by virtue of a lack of information. This is not the case for most precontemplators. Many substance abusers stay in precontemplation by doing something to keep themselves there. They minimize risks, rationalize dangers and consequences, and/or resign themselves to their addiction (DiClemente, 1991; Daniels, 1998). There is often an element of rebellion and resentment at being told that they have a problem; so, confrontation and advice generally are met with resistance. However, resistance may well be a function of the approach that the therapist takes, since confrontation breeds resistance behaviors from clients (Miller, Benefield, & Tonigan, 1993).

A more recent approach encouraged by the stages of change model has been to recognize lack of motivation as a part of the process of change and to use motivational approaches to address the needs of the precontemplator (Miller, 1985; Miller & Rollnick, 1991). Although motivation is a critical issue throughout the process of change (Miller, 1999), it is a particularly important element for moving the precontemplator and contemplator forward in this process. Respect, careful and active listening, reflecting and summarizing, and highlighting discrepancies between goals and behaviors are all part of the motivational enhancement approach (Miller, 1985; Miller, Zweben, et al., 1992; Rollnick et al., 1999). This approach has become standard in a number of programs and organizations. Many treatment programs have implemented intake procedures that include evaluating readiness to change and offering a brief motivational intervention to clients identified as least ready—primarily precontemplators and early contemplators. Clients are reassessed at the end of this intervention. When they demonstrate sufficient readiness they are given a more intensive cognitive behavioral intervention. Other programs offer a preintervention or brief motivational intervention that evaluates motivation prior to a more intensive treatment. A recently funded clinical trial (Project COMBINE; O'Malley, 2000) is evaluating a treatment that combines motivational approaches with cognitive behavioral and self-help interventions and is administered in conjunction with a pharmacological adjunct. Whether programmatically or simply as part of clinical practice, therapists need to address the motivational needs of the precontemplators. If a client were not considering change, it would be counterproductive for the therapist to start with intensive, action-oriented clinical interventions.

For clients who are actively discounting both the problem and the need to change, helping them to begin to consider change is not simple. However, within every client who does not want to consider that he or she has a drug use or drinking problem there lies a reservoir of doubt. The therapist has the task of encouraging and creating in the client thoughts that the problem perhaps is really larger than perceived by the client ("Maybe all these consequences are related to my use of cocaine," "Maybe my spouse is right"). The challenge is to tap into that reservoir of doubt so that the doubt can be turned into serious consideration of change. Providing sensitive personal feedback, reflecting concerns, examining values, and exposing clients to convincing role models or to experiences that arouse emotions and awareness can be used to expose doubt and raise personal awareness. Leading the precontemplator on a path of discovery and realization requires a sensitive, empathic, but firm guide. Techniques that raise awareness without raising resistance would obviously be the most productive (DiClemente, 1991). Many of these techniques are highlighted in motivational interviewing approaches: double-sided reflection, objective feedback, and rolling with resistance (Miller & Rollnick, 1991; Bien, Miller, & Boroughs, 1993).

The challenge for the individual therapist in each of the stages is to instigate the change processes that would move the individual to the next stage. For individuals in precontemplation, the processes of consciousness raising, self-reevaluation, environmental reevaluation, and dramatic relief are the most relevant. Table 5.1 provides a view of the strategies that could be used to engage the client in these processes and the tasks to be accomplished as a result.

There are also treatment strategies that are contraindicated for the

TABLE 5.1. Tasks and Strategies for the Precontemplation Stage

Strategies	Tasks
Values clarification	Raising awareness of problem
Normative feedback	Realization of consequences and the impact
Visiting AA meeting	of behavior on others
Couple meeting	Contrast of current life and goals
Motivational interviewing	

client in precontemplation. Unless it were being done as a planned teaching experiment, giving the precontemplator a significant action assignment would not be a good match of technique to client stage. Offering medications to curtail craving or create a negative physiological response to drinking would also be contraindicated. Medication compliance and the goal of medical management of drinking cues or consequences would be subverted without adequate motivation. Alcoholics who do not want to quit drinking have been known to learn how to drink even while taking disulfiram (Antabuse). Heroin addicts have been known to use cocaine, marijuana, and other drugs along with their methadone. Medicating the client in precontemplation is problematic (at least) and potentially harmful, since the client may then believe that no medication can help. On the other hand, these medications often are very effective when the client is properly motivated (O'Brien, 1996).

Action-oriented strategies requiring activity and commitments on the part of the client are generally not useful at this stage in the change process. The one exception is when there are significant pressures and consequences from the legal system or the employment system. Under threat of consequences, precontemplators will do what is required to fulfill the letter of the law. However, they often do not really participate in a change process but simply go through the motions. Nevertheless, the threat of consequences can help the therapist gain contact and access to the individual in precontemplation that otherwise could not happen. Therapists need to use this leverage wisely and not lose it by telling the client that he or she can leave if he or she does not want to be there. Mandated and coerced presence offers an opportunity to engage the individual in the process of change and to use the motivational strategies described above and in Table 5.1.

Contemplation Stage

Once an individual begins to consider change seriously, the focal point becomes working with the client to elucidate the pros and cons of the behavior and of change. This is not as straightforward a task as it might seem. Some therapists might simply draw a line down a sheet of paper, write at the top "pros" and "cons," and then ask the client to list all of the pros and all of the cons that come to mind. It is seldom that easy. Many of the pros as well as the cons are rather ill defined and not immediately accessible. Often when asked, substance-abusing clients provide the therapist with a long list of all the negative aspects of using because he or she expects that this is what the therapist wants to hear. Encouraging the client in contemplation to describe explicitly the good things about using drugs or drinking and how substance use serves many functions for him or her is not easy. Some of these reasons are very personal and require clients to admit how they rely on alcohol and/or other drugs to manage life. Assisting the client in exploring these issues requires attentive listening and probing, open-ended questions.

During contemplation it is useful to continue engagement in the processes of consciousness raising, self-reevaluation, and environmental reevaluation. However, instead of simply making the client aware of the consequences of the problem, the task of contemplation is a comparative one in which the client evaluates the entire decisional matrix. What is critical is whether the considerations that foster change outweigh those that do not. Table 5.2 offers a schema for these considerations.

There are self-report measures that can tap into these considerations and their relative importance. Do the reasons supporting change outweigh the reasons for resisting change? Exploring this question is not simply an exercise in reasoning. Each reason has an affective valence or weight that is important to evaluate. There may be many moderately important reasons to change and one major reason not to change, or vice versa, that would influence the decision making. It is interesting to note

TABLE 5.2. Decisional Balance Worksheet

Considerations against change	Considerations for change
Positives of the behavior	Negatives of the behavior
Negatives of the change	Positives of the change

that similar considerations appear to be relevant across different substance abuse problems and for individuals in treatment as well as those who change without formal treatment (Klingemann, 1991; Sobell, Sobell, Tonneato, & Leo, 1993; Tucker, Vuchinich, & Pukish, 1995).

Carl was a heavy drinker who had thought about his drinking and was well satisfied that there was *little* problem in his frequent drinking except that it led to nagging by his wife. One day while he was driving with his family along the freeway, his 3-year-old son pointed to a billboard advertising a particular brand of liquor and stated that is what his daddy drank and that is what he was going to drink. This experience had such an impact on Carl's thinking and decisional balance that he moved to a decision to quit drinking and smoking. Rather quickly he stopped drinking almost entirely. His fear of his son imitating his pattern of drinking was a consideration that outweighed his many positive reasons for drinking.

It is difficult to create these kinds of experiences in the therapy session. However, there are techniques that can foster reevaluation and affective arousal similar to what Carl experienced. Sometimes it is possible to have clients imagine past events that represent particularly painful or difficult consequences related to their substance abuse. For those clients with a family history, the therapist can help the client to reexperience some of the parental or familial events that were marred by drinking. The objective of these exercises is to have the client recognize and relive emotionally some important experiences that may have been glossed over. In a similar way the therapist can ask clients to imagine that they are functioning and interacting without the aid of the drug in order to begin a discussion of the pros and cons of changing the particular substance-abusing behavior. Psychodrama and exercises that were developed in gestalt therapy can also be used to make decisional considerations more vivid, affect-laden, and powerful. For example, role playing a conversation with a parent, spouse, or boss where the client moves from one chair to another in the room and takes both parts of the conversation could elicit significant self-reevaluation. The ultimate goal of such exercises is to promote the reevaluation process and the making of a firm decision to change.

Any strategies or techniques to promote decision making would be useful with the client in contemplation. Values clarification exercises where the client is asked to explore hopes and dreams, to examine what values are represented by the current lifestyle, or to remember family values taught while growing up can set the stage for decision making. Few clients had as a goal in life to become a drug abuser. Most still have some ideas about what they would like in their lives. Accessing their aspirations and currently unrealized values can encourage a serious evaluation of "where I am" versus "where I want to be or hoped to be." Many of the motivational interviewing strategies described by Miller and Rollnick (1991) are designed to address the ambivalence experienced in the contemplation stage and to promote decision making for change. Training in these strategies of amplification, double-sided reflection, and rolling with resistance can be very helpful for the therapist seeking to engender contemplation. There are also a number of books that discuss the social-psychological phenomenon of persuasion (e.g., Cialdini, 1988). These outline strategies used in marketing and other professional settings where the objective is to have a consumer consider and ultimately purchase a product or choose a service. Adapting these strategies for use in the treatment of substance use would be particularly helpful in working with the client in contemplation. In many ways the therapist with a client in the contemplation stage must be a bit of a sales person. The therapist needs to engender interest in and consideration of change and ultimately make change something the client chooses to do.

Preparation Stage

Making a decision and following through with the appropriate action are not the same. Although the primary responsibility for taking action must reside with the client, the therapist can assist in helping the client prepare for action. A serious misconception held by some therapists is the belief that once a decision is made the client moves automatically into action. Client statements like "I really am convinced that I should do something about my cocaine problem" or "I am going to quit drinking" are music to the ear of the therapist who has been working with a client in precontemplation and contemplation. However, the large number of clients who drop out of treatment early in therapy, often after making some of these statements, are a sobering reminder of the elusive nature of these decisions (Wickizer et al., 1994; Smith, Subich, & Kalodner, 1995; Simpson & Joe, 1993). The focus of treatment for the client in preparation is planning and commitment enhancement. It is the sufficiency of the plan and the strength of the commitment that will enable the client to begin to take appropriate actions and to follow through on the plan.

The treatment plan (described in Chapter 4) is not the same as the action plan. This is an important distinction. Treatment programs have settings, components, time frames, and recommendations. Being in treatment implies that the client will follow the treatment plan (e.g., attend outpatient group two times a week, one self-help group a week, a once a week meeting with an individual therapist, a family meeting once a month). Often the plan is a predetermined course that is recommended to all clients for whom this level of treatment is deemed appropriate. From the stages of change perspective, the treatment plan should serve the client's action plan. The action plan specifies what the client needs to do to change the drinking and drug use behavior. In the preparation stage, the therapist should help the client construct this action plan (DiClemente, 1991). There is some evidence from the smoking cessation literature that if there is some specificity to the action plan, such as setting a date when the action will begin, there is a greater probability of moving into the action stage (Agency for Health Care Policy and Research, 1996). Specificity in the plan promotes action.

The action plan should contain the specifics of what the client will do to quit or modify the behavior and how to handle the different days of the week and the different opportunities to use that can be anticipated. The plan also should identify who could help and how and what could go wrong, in order to build contingency plans. Table 5.3 illustrates a change plan worksheet that was used in the motivational enhancement therapy developed for Project MATCH. How detailed a plan should be depends on the needs of the client and how much support needs to be provided in terms of treatment setting and intensity. A less detailed plan in a day treatment setting is less worrisome than the same plan in regular weekly outpatient treatment. Planning, however, is not ordinarily one of the strengths of the substance abuser. Instead, immediate gratification and what Albert Ellis calls low frustration tolerance (LFT; Ellis, McInerney, & DiGiuseppe, 1988) are characteristics of many substance abusers. The therapist needs to work diligently to overcome the reluctance to plan and identify planning as one of the important elements that promote successful change and differentiate the life of sobriety from that of abusing drugs and alcohol.

Planning should include both identification of the strategies to move successfully into action and a checkup on the skills needed to implement these strategies. One of the most important contributions of the therapist to the client in preparation is to provide an evaluation of the skills needed to implement the plan and attempt to remediate any skill deficits. A plan

TABLE 5.3. Change Plan Worksheet

The changes I want to make are:

The most important reasons why I want to make these changes are:

The steps I plan to take in changing are:

The ways other people can help me are:

Person   Possible ways to help

I will know that my plan is working if:

Some things that could interfere with my plan are:

Note. From Miller, Zweben, DiClemente, and Rychtarik (1992).

that does not include anger management training for a client whose anger often triggers his or her drug use will be flawed from its inception. The skills that are needed for change can be explored by using several techniques. The most extensive procedure is called a functional analysis of the various areas of the life of the drug abuser (Carroll, 1999; Sobell & Sobell, 1981). This analysis covers all the major areas of life functioning in order to identify the factors that maintain the drug use behaviors. The objective is to discover the problematic reinforcers and lack of appropriate reinforcers that influence the behavior of the individual. The Community Reinforcement Approach, which involves setting up social events, employment groups, and other options to replace the problematic reinforcement system with a more adaptive one that is incompatible with drug use (DeLeon, Melnick, Kressel, & Jainchill, 1994; Mallams, Godley, Hall, & Meyers, 1982), is one approach that has emerged in response to the indications provided through a functional analysis of substance use. The Addiction Severity Index (ASI) was created to obtain a more comprehensive view of the needs of drug abusers and examines multiple areas of functioning that can be problematic, including dimensions of substance use and associated medical, employment, legal, family/social, and psychological problems (McLellan et al., 1994). There are intriguing data indicating that the more services that are accessed to address the various needs of the drug and alcohol abusing population, the better the outcomes (McClellan et al., 1994). More comprehensive planning for addressing the varied needs of the clients appears to improve outcomes significantly.

If more extensive methods for assessment and planning are not available, the most productive way to explore problems that interfere with change would be to examine in depth the client's past attempts to change the drug and alcohol use behavior. Previous change attempts can be very instructive. What were the plans in the prior attempts? For how long did the client succeed? What were the circumstances of the return to using? These are the same types of questions that are used to debrief a slip or relapse. The answers can offer a good view of the types of situations and challenges that the client found difficult or impossible to conquer. The skills and strategies to deal with these challenges need to be addressed in the current change plan.

Darlene was a 28-year-old cocaine addict who had a 10-year history of use that accelerated from snorting cocaine to smoking crack. The cocaine had destroyed her marriage and significantly impaired her ability to parent her 7-year-old son, who currently was being cared for by her mother. Darlene had completed high school and had several jobs as a clerk in various retail stores. She had wanted to go to college but did not have the money and was unsure what she would do with a degree. She started using drugs in high school, and the problem escalated after she graduated and became involved with a man who was selling drugs. She had easy access to drugs for a while, but after a breakup with this man, she became a prostitute as a way to support her habit. Her subsequent marriage was a bright spot, since she found a partner who wanted to take her away from her drug abusing life and to have a family. Shortly after the birth of their son, she again began to use cocaine, which created severe marital problems. At the breakup of her marriage, she returned to her drug-abusing life. Currently she was living with a man who had a serious heroin problem. On the ASI, she indicated significant problems in the areas of family, employment, alcohol, drugs, and psychological functioning. She appeared to have a moderate depression that could have been present prior to the drug abuse. When she would try to stop using cocaine, she could stay clean only for a week or two. Some problem, often a frustrating interaction with her son, her mother, her ex-husband, or her boyfriend, would get her down, and she would seek escape in her cocaine and crack use. She had no female friends except for a couple of women she knew from her days as a prostitute. She had a sexually transmitted disease and was very concerned about contracting AIDS. She realized that this lifestyle was not working, and she came into the treatment center determined to change her life and get away from her cocaine habit.

Although one would need a more detailed exploration in each of these areas, it is clear from this thumbnail sketch that the action plan for Darlene should be multifaceted and comprehensive if it is to have a chance of success. Strategies and skills to deal with depression, relationships, employment, parenting, and family relations are pertinent to a viable action plan that will increase her ability to sustain abstinence beyond the 1 or 2 weeks that she had been able to achieve in the past. The action plan has to include where she will live, how she will handle her current relationship, who will support sobriety, alternative ways to manage frustration, and dealing with other drug-use-related cues and problems. In addition, financial support, employment, and contacts between her and her mother and son would be important problem areas to address both in the action plan and in the treatment plan.

Commitment enhancement is the other critical task of the preparation stage, although most addiction therapists are not given much training in it. Motivation and commitment are the responsibility of the client and not the therapist. However, there are ways that the therapist can support and enhance the client's commitment. Choice increases commitment (Prochaska & DiClemente, 1984). Making sure that the client makes choices among possible alternative elements in his or her action or treatment plan can increase a sense of commitment. Encouraging words about the client's ability to change as well as recalling past efforts that were successful can increase the sense of efficacy and choice. Imagining success, as some world-class gymnasts and skaters do prior to a performance, can also enhance commitment. Denigrating ability or focusing on past failures would do the opposite. Encouraging positive self-talk similar to that in the children's story of "The Little Engine That Could" also could be helpful if based on realistic views of skills and problems. Posing potential barriers to change so the client can practice verbally how to overcome these barriers can also be used to create better-prepared coping strategies. Helping the client remove any last vestiges of the ambivalence that interferes with action can also be viewed as commitment-enhancing. Commitment is needed to negotiate the action plan, particularly in the early phases of action, where the discomfort, sense of loss, disorientation, and physiological reactions are the strongest.

Action Stage

Once the action plan is designed and the commitment to follow through with the plan shored up, the individual enters the action stage. The preceding sequence may sound idealistic, since many clients move into action before a plan is formulated or move into action in fits and starts. What we are describing is an ideal path of movement through the stages of change. However, the tasks of each stage remain important regardless of how the action is begun. One way or another, the successful solution of these tasks is critical to effective action and long-term change.

The need for commitment in the early part of the action stage is paramount, since there is much pain and no apparent gain in the first steps of breaking the addiction and removing the drug from the system physically and psychologically. Clients need hope of future relief and a strong desire to break the addiction in order to sustain the effort needed in the action stage. The action plan needs to be implemented, reviewed regularly, and revised as needed. It is the unusual planning process that does not encounter some unanticipated problems once the plan is undertaken. This is as true for building a house as it is for changing behaviors. Some expected support may not be forthcoming, drug-using networks may exert more pressure than anticipated, or a drug-using spouse may be very threatened. All of these can create a crisis that requires additional problem solving and alternative strategies in the revision of the plan. Review and revision are important tasks in early action that continue into the maintenance stage.

In some respects the therapist has less to do in the action stage when the client is working the agreed-upon plan. Like the coach who prepares the players for the game but can do little once the game has begun, the therapist can offer encouragement and support and provide guidance and strategies along the way (DiClemente, 1991). However, it is up to the players to complete the plays. It is the shifting from more cognitive and experiential processes to the behavioral processes of counterconditioning, stimulus control, and reinforcement management that is the central task to be accomplished by the client (Perz, DiClemente, & Carbonari, 1996). The latter processes need to be used to promote abstinence and to cope with urges. The therapist should assist the client in building strategies that incorporate these processes. Creating alternative reinforcers and responses for cues to use, offering relaxation training, refusal skills training, assertiveness and positive communication training, and helping the client avoid cues that cannot be tolerated are part of the action preparation that enables the client to succeed.

Orchestrating the elements in the action plan to mesh with the various types of treatments and interventions available to meet the needs of the client is a second important function for the individual therapist or counselor. The adage espoused by some self-help groups to not get involved in any other type of treatment or other stressful activities until the addict has one year of sobriety has an understandable basis. However, it is not a good rule for all and possibly not helpful for many clients (DiClemente, Carbonari, & Velasquez, 1992). Some couple treatment, family therapy, anxiety and anger management, pharmacotherapy, job skills training, additional education, or other adjunctive interventions should be worked into the mix as the client moves through the action stage (Roth & Fonagy, 1996). The objective is to sustain successful action with regard to changing the alcohol- and drug-abusing behaviors for a long enough period of time to gain some stability so the client can move into the maintenance stage. Solving associated problems can assist in creating successful sustained action to abstain from drugs that needs to continue for at least 3 to 6 months before entry into the maintenance stage.

For some clients, pharmacotherapy is an important and valuable part of the action plan. There are active programs of research being sponsored by the National Institute on Alcohol Abuse and Alcoholism and by the National Institute on Drug Abuse to develop medications that can help individuals to stop drinking and using drugs (Egertson, Fox, & Leshner, 1997; Barber & O'Brien, 1999). These medications focus on replacing an abused substance with a safer one (methadone maintenance, nicotine replacement), interfering with a drug's mechanism of action to dampen its effect or lessen the craving (naltrexone, acamprosate), or creating a reaction that would make taking the drug less attractive (disulfiram) (see Carroll, 1996a). Each of these types of medications can offer some assistance in breaking the habit pattern and allow the individual time to institute alternate patterns of behavior. However, it is important to note that these medications most often have been tested in combination with a behavioral or psychological treatment program. Engaging in the behavioral treatment in addition to taking the medication is usually the pattern that produces the significant effect. Note that most of these medications are not designed to be taken for extended periods. Ultimately the important behavioral tasks required to complete the action and maintenance stages successfully will need to be accomplished so that removal of the medication does not provoke relapse.

Maintenance Stage

Few clients remain in treatment as they enter the maintenance stage of change unless the focus of the individual therapy has shifted successfully to encompass a broader spectrum of client problems beyond those related to the substance use. (Therapeutic communities are the significant exception to this rule since they usually require a stay of many months or even years.) This loss of contact during the maintenance stage is understandable. Once clients have successfully modified their substance abuse behavior, they reach a plateau of smoother road after the long climb up the mountain of the action stage of change. However, lack of contact during the maintenance stage is unfortunate since recovery from an addiction represents the stabilization of what generally had been a chronic condition. This stabilization takes time and requires effort and vigilance. For the most part this lack of follow-up contact is due to a failure on the part of both therapist and client to define the specific tasks of maintenance. Often expectations about how therapy can help during maintenance are unclear and/or limited.

The tasks of maintenance are to sustain change over time and to integrate that change into the lifestyle of the individual so that the new behavior, abstinence from drugs, becomes the preferred habitual behavior of that individual. Sustaining change requires meeting successfully any challenges that arise to threaten the decision to change or the path of change. Relapse after a long period of abstinence often follows one of two predictable paths (Marlatt & Gordon, 1985; Brownell et al., 1986). The first is when the client becomes somewhat overconfident in his or her ability to control drug use. The second involves the erosion of the commitment to quit using, often fueled by disillusionment with the sober life experienced after change. Many in the first group of clients are convinced that they will be able stop again without much trouble. For the latter group of individuals there often is a decision, either partially or well formed, to return to the substance. In both cases the individuals decide to use or fail to avoid drinking or using drugs once or several times. This return to use compromises maintenance of abstinence and threatens to undermine previous progress toward sustained change. The problem for the individual therapist in this stage is to decide how and when to work with the client over the long haul in order to be able to help with the insidious processes and events that threaten change during this stage.

Individual therapy can respond well to the needs of clients in the maintenance stage if it is flexible and broadly focused. Maintenance is the most productive time to work on the multiple problems that contributed to the development of the addiction or that remain as consequences of the years of abuse. Resolving marital conflicts, long-standing beliefs that undermine self-esteem and confidence, fears and anxieties, and past abuse or familial problems are important targets of longer-term treatment of the substance abuser. Managed care's reluctance to support longer-term care is shortsighted since the resolution of these problems brings with it more stable change as well as healthier and more productive citizens (Finney, Moos, & Timko, 1999; McLellan et al., 1994; Moos, Finney, & Cronkite, 1990; Vaillant, 1995). Individual treatment is ideal in the maintenance stage since it can be designed to occur at less frequent intervals and to include one or more associated goals beyond sobriety. For individuals who are doing well at resolving associated problems with minimal assistance, some type of office checkup schedule, similar to dental hygiene visits, may suffice. Follow-up visits would enable the therapist to meet once every 2 months with the client to see how things are going and whether there is any need for more assistance or access to resources. The function of the individual session in this case would be different. The checkup visit could consist of continuing the reinforcement of the decision and path to sobriety, problem solving any remaining issues, and examining any threat to sobriety.

Medications for other psychiatric problems and adjunctive therapy or services often are useful in assisting the client in making the changes in drug and alcohol behavior permanent. The individual therapist must avoid the problematic belief that he or she can help the client with every need or problem. Having an extensive list of resources where the client can obtain assistance in resume writing and job interviewing, be evaluated for medication for ongoing medical or psychological problems, receive family therapy, or seek social security and other benefits is very important. Active referral with support is an important therapy skill during the maintenance stage. Finding out exactly what services the client can get at a particular agency and how to access those resources is part of the therapist's responsibility. Helping the client realize the need for and the commitment to following through are also important elements in the treatment of clients in the maintenance stage. Finally, checking to see how the referral went and whether there is a need to reevaluate the referral represents another important task for the individual therapist with a client in maintenance.

Referral to self-help groups provides access to an important support system that individuals can use to help them successfully negotiate the maintenance stage (Longabaugh, Wirtz, Beattie, Noel, & Stout, 1995; Velasquez, Carbonari, & DiClemente, 1999). These groups (e.g., Alcoholics Anonymous, Rational Recovery, Women for Sobriety) can provide ubiquitous access and support when an individual needs an assist in meeting challenges and problems that threaten sobriety. There is an interesting new twist to these groups with the advent of technology. Access to self-help or mutual assistance groups through the Internet is becoming more popular and can provide a level of support that is even more readily available than the traditional meeting (Nowinski, 1999).

However, self-help and mutual support are not sufficient for some clients. This is particularly true for those who have associated psychopathology or who have serious skill deficits. More intensive individual and/or group treatments may be necessary to assist them in creating a new lifestyle and in resolving related problems. In this case individual treatment becomes a primary vehicle for assisting the client in addressing psychological distress and symptoms, discovering and promoting alternative reinforcing activities and behaviors, developing and refining appropriate skills, and problem solving situations that pose dangers to sobriety and health.

Relapse and Recycling

The return to substance abuse is a discouraging event for client and therapist. Even the single use of a substance after some period of abstinence can create a strain on the therapeutic relationship. To move forward in the process of change both the therapist and the client need to be invested in achieving successful, lasting change in the drinking and drug use behaviors. A slip or lapse raises many questions about the stability of the change and the dedication of the client. Suspicions, guilt, recriminations, and doubt are the normal responses to the violation of abstinence after a sustained period of change. If not checked, these feelings can create an atmosphere conducive to decreased motivation and set the stage for a more robust return to the substance use (Brownell et al., 1986). A relapse or more complete return to the substance abusing behaviors increases the intensity of the emotions and reactions described above. It is this insidious process that can undermine the therapeutic bond and create distance between therapist and client at precisely the time when they need to be working together to manage this threat to successful change. The therapist must set the stage for working together during this difficult time while, at the same time, avoiding messages that predict or promote a relapse. This is a delicate and difficult task. We address the issue of relapse in considerable detail in Chapter 9. In this section, we highlight some of the most relevant clinical issues related to relapse, from a stages of change perspective, along with associated clinical responses.

If the therapist can create an atmosphere in which the client feels comfortable coming into the treatment setting to discuss the slip or relapse, the work of the individual therapy is clear. In this regard, the key tasks are to isolate and contain the substance use behavior, reinstate the commitment and decision to continue with the change, counter discouragement and depression, address the cognitive and behavioral triggers that are operating, and support reengagement in the process of change (Carroll, 1996b). For the individual who is slipping back and beginning to return to the former pattern of problem behavior, rapid action to help the client get back into action, to revise the action plan to address the slip, and to encourage and support are the most important tasks. If the slips have turned into a more significant relapse or collapse, the goals of the therapist's work with the client are to ensure that he or she becomes a recycler (Prochaska et al., 1992).

Normalizing the process of relapse without creating a self-fulfilling prophecy is a significant challenge. Probably the most useful way to do this is to interpret relapse as an important step on the road to recovery and as part of the process of change. Race car drivers and their pit crews learn from every race how to improve the car, increase the speed, and develop strategies that make winning the race more probable. Talented basketball players continue to practice in order to raise the level of their game. Recounting how Larry Bird and Michael Jordan were always the last ones to leave practice after having a sub-par game or in preparation for a playoff game can serve as instructive examples to cite to clients who believe that they should be perfectly successful from the start.

Rather than dwelling on relapse when it occurs, the therapist would do better to focus on recycling. Learning from past attempts to change and then reevaluating where the individual is in the process of change are productive tasks for the client in relapse and his or her therapist. Some individuals are so discouraged and become so lacking in hope that they move back into precontemplation and refuse for the present to consider another change attempt. Others return to the ambivalence of the contemplation stage and consider the possibility of another attempt but not immediately. Still others are like the rider who falls off the horse and wants to get back on as soon as possible. These individuals move back to preparation for another change attempt and are immediately planning the next attempt. However, in our experience, movement from a relapse that either represents an almost complete return to the former habit pattern and precontemplation or recycling back into another quick attempt at action are less frequent than a return to contemplation. After a significant attempt to change a behavior that fails badly, the individual seems to need some time to regroup and get ready for another attempt. This is part of the reason that changing addictive behaviors takes such a long time both at an individual and at a macro level.

Assessing where the individual has landed after the relapse is the first step to reorganizing the goals and strategies of treatment. The therapist needs to evaluate what went wrong both with the treatment plan and with the client's action plan. What were the elements of each of these plans that did not work? What ancillary treatments or resources were needed that were not provided? What unanticipated people, places, or things interfered with the plan? Was there a letdown in commitment, a deficit in skills, or some other problem that led to the collapse of the action plan? Problem solving at this point should look at the entire process of change and determine if there were tasks at various stages of change that were not sufficiently addressed or accomplished. For example, if the decisional balance was only slightly tilted toward action or the positive reasons for engaging in the substance abuse not countered adequately, work remains to be done with the client's decision making. The answer to the above questions can redirect the focus of the treatment to the appropriate stage and strategies.

PLACING INDIVIDUAL THERAPY IN A
PROCESS OF CHANGE PERSPECTIVE

The process of change is always greater than the formal interventions delivered by the therapist. In fact, multiple interventions and treatments often contribute to the process of successful change for any single substance abuser. In Project MATCH almost 50% of the outpatients and over 50% of the aftercare clients had had a previous inpatient treatment for substance abuse (Project MATCH Research Group, 1997a). Prior treatment contributed in some way to the work of the Project MATCH therapists, who saw the clients for 12 weeks of individual outpatient or aftercare treatment. This is an important reality to remember. In the best-case scenario, the therapist and the intervention contribute to the client's movement through the process of change or support the change the client is already making (Tucker, Vuchinich, & Pukish, 1995). However, treatments or therapists are never completely responsible for the change in the substance abuse behavior. Most often therapists are not present to view the entire process of change for a particular client. Sometimes therapists are fortunate enough to be with a client long enough to see the ultimate positive outcome. For each therapist there are a few clients who have made significant and lasting changes and who either remain in treatment or return to therapy after a time to thank the therapist for changing their lives. However, there are many more who drop out of treatment or leave treatment appearing not to have changed much. Precious little is known about their outcomes. When we look at the research evaluating long-term outcomes for substance abuse clients, it is clear that many who go to treatment programs do well (Moos et al., 1990; Finney, Moos, & Timko, 1999; Vaillant, 1995; Project MATCH Research Group, 1998a). However, research also has demonstrated that even some of the dropouts from treatment are able to change and succeed in recovering from alcohol and drug problems (DiClemente & Scott, 1997). Ultimate client change may not necessarily occur within the context of a single dose of individual therapy.

For most clients the individual therapist assists them in moving along the path to change without ever seeing the ultimate outcome of the process of change. This is particularly true in individual therapy. Because of cost and the time involved in providing the individual focus, clients are often anxious to know when they can finish therapy. Some simply stop when they believe that they have had enough treatment. In the ideal world, it would be preferable if clients chose a single therapist and continued to work with that therapist until he or she reached successful, maintained change of the substance abuse problem, no matter how long that process took. Then the therapist could assist clients in moving through the stages of change, help with relapse and recycling through these stages, and finally support the maintenance of change until the client reached sustained change of the substance abuse problem. However, with some few exceptions, this is not how treatment works. Most often treatment is episodic and delivered by a sequence of different programs and therapists. It is only when a single therapist or program has a vision of the entire process of change that they can see more clearly the role that they are playing for this particular client in this process of change. Each therapy experience can advance or hinder movement through the process of change. A therapist, who may have the opportunity to see a client only for a single session or for a more substantial period of time, has the responsibility to provide an experience that fosters client engagement in the process of change. For the therapist thoughtful, skillful, and respectful of this process, individual therapy can be the catalyst to move that individual through an important part of the journey through this process of change.

SUMMARY

• Individual treatment is uniquely suited to the concepts of the stages of change model.

• The initial task of individual treatment is assessing where the individual stands in the process of changing his or her substance use.

• It is important to assess the client's stage of change on an ongoing basis, as individuals can move from one stage to the next from week to week, or even day to day.

• Individual sessions with a client in precontemplation permit the therapist to explore the reasons why this individual entered treatment as well as ways to move him or her from precontemplation. An approach encouraged by the stages of change model has been to recognize lack of motivation as a part of the process of change and to use motivational approaches to address the needs of the precontemplator.

• When a client begins to seriously contemplate change, the focus shifts to working with the client to elucidate the pros and cons of the behavior of change. Strategies to promote decision making are useful in working with the client in contemplation.

- Clients do not necessarily move into action once a decision to change has been made. Instead, they often move into a stage of preparation, where the focus is on planning and commitment enhancement.

- Once the action plan is designed and the commitment to follow through with the plan has developed, the individual enters the action stage.

- The tasks of maintenance are to sustain change over time and to integrate that change into the lifestyle of the individual so that the new behavior, abstinence from drugs, becomes the preferred, habitual behavior of the individual.

- Relapses, when they occur, can be discouraging events, for both the client and the therapist. It is important for the therapist to create an atmosphere where the client feels comfortable coming into a session to discuss a slip or relapse.

6

GROUP TREATMENT

A wide and heterogeneous range of therapeutic interventions, including almost every major psychological and psychiatric treatment strategy, have been tried with substance abusers (Miller, 1992; Miller et al., 1995). These approaches differ on a number of dimensions, such as their general philosophical orientation (e.g., disease or behavioral), treatment setting (e.g., inpatient or outpatient), and specific intervention modalities (e.g., individual, family, marital, or group therapy) (Institute of Medicine, 1990; Miller, 1992; Miller and Hester, 1986). Among the possible therapeutic modalities, group therapy has emerged as one of the most widely used—if not the modal form of—treatment or therapy delivery within the realm of addictions rehabilitation (Golden, Khantzian, & McAuliffe, 1994; Levy, 1997; Miller & Hester, 1980; Stinchfield, Owen, & Winters, 1994).

GROUP VERSUS INDIVIDUAL TREATMENT

Individual therapy in general, and more specifically with substance abusers, has a number of benefits that promote its use (Rounsaville & Carroll, 1997), and we described some of these in Chapter 5. When compared to other therapeutic approaches, individual therapy appears to include the following relative benefits: (1) it provides privacy and confidentiality, enabling the individual to discuss sensitive issues more openly; (2) it provides an individualized pace, allowing the therapist more flexibility in addressing the client's problems as they arise over the course of therapy; (3) a greater percentage of time is spent on the individual's problem in comparison to group therapy, again allowing more individual tailoring of the therapy session around the client's concerns; and (4) the structure of individual therapy may have advantages in dealing with certain types of problems (e.g., relationship issues) or individuals (e.g., those with personality disorders) (Rounsaville & Carroll, 1997).

Despite the potential benefits of individual therapy, Stinchfield, Owen, and Winters (1994) indicate that group therapy is the most common form of treatment for substance abusers. It has surpassed individual therapy as the psychotherapeutic treatment of choice and is used in nearly all outpatient substance abuse programs in the United States (R. H. Price, Burke, et al., 1991). Group therapy is thought to be an essential component of an integrated, individualized approach to the treatment of substance use disorders (Kaufman, 1994).

A number of factors have contributed to the widespread use of group therapy in the treatment of substance abusers. A particularly important economic factor in this age of managed care and cost containment is that group therapy is less costly than individual therapy. Rounsaville and Carroll (1997) indicate that most groups typically have at least six members and may have two therapists, thus leading to at least a tripling of the number of clients per therapy hour over individual therapy. Miller and Hester (1980) noted that the primary advantage of group is in the area of cost-effectiveness.

However, potential cost savings are not the only reason that group approaches have assumed prominence within substance abuse treatment programs. It may be appropriate to distinguish between group therapy as a form of treatment delivery and as a type of treatment. As a type of treatment, a number of approaches to group therapy have been promoted for dealing with substance abusers, and a number of curative factors associated with the group process identified (e.g., Brown & Yalom, 1977; Flores, 1988; Rogers & McMillin, 1989; Vinogradov & Yalom, 1989). From the perspective of group as a treatment delivery format, a number of different types of interventions, ranging from highly structured social skills training to less structured interpersonal and interactive approaches, are delivered in group settings.

CURATIVE FACTORS OPERATIVE
IN GROUP TREATMENT

The use of a group delivery format capitalizes on the operation of a number of "curative factors" associated with groups as a form of treatment (Flores, 1988; Yalom, 1995). A number of features of group therapy are thought to contribute to the behavior change process (Kaufman, 1994), including the following:

• Many of the problems or skill deficits associated with substance abuse are interpersonal in nature, and the context of a group provides a realistic yet "safe" setting for practice in the acquisition or refinement of new social skills (Chaney, 1989; Flores, 1988; Monti, Abrams, Kadden, & Cooney, 1989).

• Important aspects of social skills training treatment, particularly modeling, rehearsal, and feedback, occur more powerfully in a group setting (Chaney, 1989; Rugel, 1991).

• A number of features of group approaches, including the instillation of hope that it is possible to overcome a substance use problem, the imparting of information, the realization that others share similar problems, altruism or helping others with their problems, the development of socializing techniques, the modeling of appropriate behaviors, and the development and enhancement of interpersonal learning and trust, appear to produce cognitive, affective, and behavioral changes (Brown & Yalom, 1977; Flores, 1988; Yalom, 1995).

• Peer feedback in the context of a therapy group provides an opportunity to observe and "confront" others' and one's own "denial system" either directly or indirectly through identification and modeling (Golden et al., 1994; Stinchfield et al., 1994; Washton, 1992).

• A client model whose skill level is only somewhat greater than that of the observer is likely to have more impact on behavior than a therapist serving as a model. Rehearsal with and feedback from peers is likely to be more realistic than in individual treatment and may also serve to produce generalizability of the behavior change.

• Groups provide clients the opportunity to change their social networks, resulting in the development of a meaningful support system that will further enhance the recovery process.

• The group supports and directs an individual towards a commitment to recovery. This commitment is a fundamental ingredient in the process of behavior change and in the process of achieving and maintaining an alcohol- and drug-free lifestyle (N. S. Miller, 1995)

Data support the importance of a number of these curative factors from a client's perspective (Lovejoy et al., 1995). Methadone maintenance clients who had successfully completed a relapse prevention group that they were required to attend because of continued cocaine use were asked about those factors that they found helpful in their successfully completing the group. Over 70% of the clients rated their group therapy sessions as especially important. Over the course of the group they found that they were not "alone" in dealing with their problems but that other group members had similar experiences, that they were able to talk openly about their addiction in a safe and supportive environment without experiencing feelings of shame and loneliness, and that the feelings of closeness and camaraderie that developed among the clients were particularly important for them. Similarly, Lovett and Lovett (1991) found that assuming personal responsibility for one's behavior, overcoming isolation, increasing self-understanding, and experiencing a sense of group cohesiveness were the most valued factors in the group therapy experience of alcoholics involved in an inpatient treatment program.

ADAPTING THE STAGES OF CHANGE
MODEL OF BEHAVIOR CHANGE
TO A GROUP TREATMENT FORMAT

Rounsaville and Carroll (1997) have noted that almost all major schools of individual psychotherapy have been adapted to a group format. This also applies to the stages of change model. As exemplified in Chapter 5, the model lends itself to individualized interventions, given its focus on the individual's readiness to change and the use of a number of interventions that target the individual's decision-making process and those processes of change that accompany a given stage of readiness. A practical question is whether therapeutic interventions consistent with the stages of change model, given its highly individualized focus, can be translated successfully into a group therapy format. Data from recent studies suggest that this translation is possible.

Annis, Schober, and Kelly (1996) have developed an intervention model in which components of a structured relapse prevention model (e.g., assessment of high-risk drinking situations, motivational interviewing, individual treatment plan, acquisition of relapse prevention skills, and maintenance counseling) are targeted to the stage of readiness for change that an individual client is in. Graham, Annis, Brett, and Venesoen (1996) investigated the extent to which such targeted intervention strategies that have been developed with individual therapy as a focus could be generalized and successfully implemented in a group setting. They compared a structured relapse prevention program delivered either as individual therapy or as group therapy with concurrent brief individual sessions. The two conditions resulted in similar levels of attendance and client satisfaction, and no differences were found in drinking-related outcome measures at a 12-month follow-up. The only difference at follow-up was in the area of social support from friends, which favored the group therapy format. The results of Graham et al. (1996) suggest that it is possible to transfer successfully from individual therapy to a group therapy format.

Kaufman (1994) notes that both individual and group therapy approaches have merit and provide different benefits and that, as such, attempts should be made to integrate their use in treating substance abusers. Such a suggestion has been supported by the work of Hoffman et al. (1994). These investigators found that retention and treatment exposure of cocaine-abusing clients could be enhanced either by providing more frequent and intensive groups or by combining group therapy with individual services. Given this backdrop, it is not surprising to see the increased focus on incorporating the stages of change model and motivational enhancement techniques into therapy groups that are delivered either as stand-alone groups or integrated with individual therapy (e.g., Amrod, 1997; Barrie, 1991; Rugel, 1991; Yu & Watkins, 1996).

Before describing such group approaches, we will examine some of the logistical, practical, and conceptual issues that must be considered in developing a group approach.

"OPEN" VERSUS "CLOSED" GROUPS

A number of issues concerning the nature and composition of the group need to be taken into account when attempting to translate individual therapy principles into a group therapy format. The first is whether the group will be "open," which suggests that new members will be added to an ongoing group across time, or "closed," indicating that a single cohort of clients enters the group together and continues together without the infusion of new members. There are examples of each of these approaches in the literature dealing with the application of the stages of change model to group therapy (e.g., Barrie, 1991; Yu & Watkins, 1996).

This distinction has a number of logistical issues tied to it, such as the need to develop a sufficient pool of clients to begin a cohort and what to do with such clients while they are awaiting entry into the group. Closed groups may benefit more from group-related curative factors, such as cohesion and the development of interpersonal trust, because of the ongoing involvement of the same clients across time. In contrast, open groups may be more frequently diverted from substantive issues as they work to assimilate new members into the group. A related issue is determining the optimal size of the group. It is important to have a "critical mass" of clients remaining in closed groups after members have dropped out. On the other hand, open groups may have to limit entry into the group so that new members can be assimilated without the group process becoming overly destabilized.

HOMOGENEOUS VERSUS HETEROGENEOUS GROUP COMPOSITION

A second and somewhat related issue is whether the group should be homogeneous or heterogeneous with respect to a number of client characteristics, such as drug of choice and/or stage of readiness for change. N. S. Miller (1995) has argued for a heterogeneous group composition. He suggests that group therapy for addictions is most productively suited to including clients who are in various stages of treatment and recovery and who have different levels of treatment acceptance or resistance, motivation, and drugs of abuse. In this way clients early in treatment, struggling to become alcohol- and drug-free, will be participating in therapy groups with individuals who have been substance-free for longer periods of time and are dealing with a substance-free lifestyle. Vannicelli (1992) also advocates for heterogeneity with respect to levels of abstinence or stage of recovery. Having members with mixed levels of abstinence can provide a sense of hope and optimism to the newly recovering member. Members will be exposed to the fact that some are able to prevent relapse and that many of those who do lapse are able to recover and continue on in the group. Similarly, Washton (1992) has noted that heterogeneous groups have the potential of enhancing the richness of the group experience and making it possible to integrate a wider variety of new members into the group. New group members are likely to find it easier to integrate themselves into a group in which they can identify readily with at least one other member.

Both Vannicelli (1992) and N. S. Miller (1995) implicitly endorse an "open" model of group membership, suggesting that the interactions between newly arrived clients and those who have been in treatment longer can be of therapeutic advantage to both. In this model of mixed-recovery group membership, clients generally join a group in early phases of recovery and continue as long as it is productive and therapeutic for them; membership is not time-limited (Vannicelli, 1992). Newer clients who are early in treatment learn a number of things from those who are more advanced in recovery, such as their not being alone or unique in their addiction, learning that treatment works, hearing others speak openly about how withdrawal symptoms diminished over time, and learning how the self-help 12-step programs can be incorporated into an abstinent lifestyle (N. S. Miller, 1995).

In contrast to this position, others have argued for homogeneous group composition (e.g., Barrie, 1991; Levy, 1997). Having a common purpose and similar goals, as well as sharing a number of common characteristics, is important for group formation, maintenance, and cohesion. Washton (1992) has suggested the principle of "maximum tolerable heterogeneity," which states that as a general rule the composition of a group should be neither too heterogeneous nor too homogeneous. Consistent with this principle, Stinchfield et al. (1994) have suggested that group therapists may need to make decisions about accepting or retaining an individual in the group on the basis not only of the individual's needs but also the needs of the group as a whole.

PHASE OF RECOVERY AND GROUP FOCUS

As presented by Barrie (1991), the issue of homogeneity versus heterogeneity appears to be related to the phase of development of the therapy group, the phase of recovery that clients are in, and the primary tasks associated with the different phases (Martin, Giannandrea, Rogers, & Johnson, 1996; Vinogradov & Yalom, 1989). Kaufman and Reoux (1988) describe three phases of recovery: achieving sobriety, early recovery, and advanced recovery. The apparent focus and goals of groups with individuals in the first two phases (achieving sobriety and early recovery) differ from those of ongoing recovery groups. In early recovery, the group focus is often on "confronting denial," increasing the individual's awareness about substance use, accepting that one has a problem requiring change, and supporting the early acquisition and maintenance of abstinence. Groups for those in advanced recovery focus on interpersonal learning to improve interpersonal relationships and the maintenance of ongoing abstinence (Vinogradov & Yalom, 1989). From the perspective of the stages of change model, these three phases of group development appear to represent the precontemplation and contemplation stages (achieving sobriety), the action stage (early recovery), and the maintenance and relapse stages (advanced recovery).

Barrie (1991) notes that difficulties often arise in the group setting when participants' aims and needs are widely divergent, which typically occurs when people from very different stages in the recovery process are mixed together in a group. Members who think that their drinking or drug use is not a problem may feel threatened and behave disruptively in a group where the majority have decided to change their drinking behavior. Similarly, the group might feel threatened by or angry at members who have not yet committed to change and who may be perceived as "in denial" or not trying. Given that individuals may be at different stages, the group interventions should address a particular stage rather than take everyone.

Because of the differing goals, the use of separate groups for clients in early recovery and for those who have been abstinent longer has been advocated (Barrie, 1991; Levy, 1997; Straussner, 1997; Vannicelli, 1992). Groups for clients earlier in recovery, analogous to the precontemplation and contemplation stages of change, share the common feature that all members have problems with substance dependence (Levy, 1997). While group members may not be fully committed or ready to stop drinking or using drugs or to enter treatment, they should at least be willing to learn about the process of addiction and the steps involved in the recovery process.

Early phase groups are most often didactic and psychoeducational in nature, frequently combining lectures, videos, and discussions among the participants (Galanter, Castaneda, & Franco, 1991; Thoreson & Budd, 1987). Informational groups provide an opportunity to increase the individual's problem awareness, solidify the commitment to behavior change and/or treatment, and obtain the cooperation and support from family members in the treatment process (Golden et al., 1994; Thoreson & Budd, 1987). Such groups are often seen as the first step in a more comprehensive treatment program (Martin et al., 1996; Straussner, 1997).

As noted previously, groups for clients in later recovery more commonly focus on interpersonal learning to improve interpersonal relationships, the maintenance of ongoing abstinence, and relapse prevention (Vinogradov & Yalom, 1989). More traditional interactional/interpersonal therapy groups are employed with such individuals (Flores, 1988; Vannicelli, 1982; Vinogradov & Yalom, 1989). Such groups focus on identifying, exploring, and attempting to resolve individual and interpersonal concerns and issues (Thoreson & Budd, 1987). The focus of such groups might also include specific behaviors or mood states, the development of insight into one's behaviors, the ability to tolerate negative moods without substance use, and the development of social support (Galanter et al., 1991).

DEVELOPING A MOTIVATIONALLY ENHANCING GROUP ATMOSPHERE

Regardless of the type of group format being used, it is important to establish a group atmosphere and culture that motivates behavior change. To a large extent this culture represents an interaction between the type of group and the professional and personal style of the group therapist(s).

Therapist Style

Cartwright (1987) indicates that an important dimension in group therapy is the extent to which the therapist/leader dominates the group. Some groups seem to be totally dominated by the leader, who defines the group's activities and their values, with all communication flowing through the leader. A number of authors have suggested that such a style is not particularly well received or useful in groups dealing with substance abuse. Rather, the ideal style for a leader conducting a group for substance abusers has been described as one in which the focus is group-oriented rather than leader-determined and in which the leader not only is knowledgeable about substance abuse but also acts as a facilitator of interpersonal process (Cartwright, 1987; Galanter et al., 1991). The maximum benefit is gained by clients when the therapy involves active partici-pation and interaction among members rather than when the group leader is domineering and controlling (Yu & Watkins, 1996). An open and more democratic group leader is likely to lead group participants to more self-exploration of substance use problems and create a sense of group cohesion.

Conducting therapy with substance abusers has often involved a somewhat confrontive style, thought to be necessary to break down the individual's defenses, particularly denial, and to convince clients to accept a long-term abstinence-oriented treatment plan (e.g., Kofoed, 1997). Yu and Watkins (1996) indicate that such an aggressive, confrontational ther-apist style is not viable in working with substance abusers. In this regard, Matano and Yalom (1991) note that an overly confrontational style in the group, in an attempt to break through "denial," can be counter-therapeutic, causing the client to leave treatment or become noncompli-ant. Rather, a more supportive and empathic approach by the counselor should be the intervention of choice (Matano & Yalom, 1991; Obert, Rawson, & Miotto, 1997; Yu & Watkins, 1996). This recommendation is consistent with the results found by Miller et al. (1993) in individual therapy. In contrast to a supportive client-centered approach based on motivational interviewing, a directive, confrontational therapist style, characteristic of more traditional approaches to substance abuse treat-ment, yielded significantly more "resistance" from clients, which in turn predicted poorer outcomes. The more the therapist confronted, the more the client(s) drank.

Group Atmosphere

The amount and nature of the psychological support offered by a group to its members is another important factor affecting the therapy process (Cartwright, 1987). Support in this context refers to the group's willing-ness to accept and encourage its members "where they are" with respect to their acknowledgment of their substance abuse problem or their stage of readiness to change. This approach differs considerably from the more traditional confrontive model where the client's unwillingness to accept the group or leader's perspective is interpreted as denial.

The incorporation of the characteristics of motivational interview-ing style (Miller & Rollnick, 1991), namely reflectiveness, therapeutic warmth, support, and empathy, appears to contribute significantly to the group atmosphere (Amrod, 1997; van Bilsen & van Emst, 1986). A similar pattern in regard to therapist style has been found in group therapy approaches with smokers (Hajek, Belcher, & Stapleton, 1985) and with alcoholics (Ends & Page, 1957). Clients involved in groups that were "group-oriented" or "client-centered," in contrast to those that were "therapist-oriented," tended to have better outcomes. Therapist authenticity, characterized by directness, acceptance, empathy, respect, self-disclosure, a nonjudgmental attitude, honesty, and openness to suggestion, appears to be one of the key principles underlying an effective group (Milgram & Rubin, 1992). Such a style would appear useful and appropriate regardless of the substance abused or whether the goals of the group are restricted to changing drug use behaviors or involve broader interpersonal and intrapersonal issues. As an example of this, van Bilsen and van Emst (1986) have described the development of a "motivational milieu therapy" in a methadone maintenance clinic. The milieu was characterized by a humanistic philosophy, an open and permissive climate in which clients were treated like adults having responsibility for themselves, and in which the staff utilized motivational interviewing techniques to increase the motivation of clients for changing their drug use behavior

STAGE-BASED GROUP APPROACHES

Recently there has been an increased focus on group therapy approaches that are based on the stages of change model and the use of motivational enhancement approaches (Amrod, 1997; Barrie, 1991; Falkowski, 1996; Yu & Watkins, 1996). These approaches have dealt with a number of the previously described therapeutic and logistical issues somewhat differently. Yu and Watkins (1996) have developed a group approach for individuals mandated into treatment for a driving while intoxicated offense. Their approach represents a closed group in which clients are involved as cohorts that continue together moving through advancing stages of change. In contrast, Barrie (1991) suggests having a separate group for substance abusers who are in the precontemplation stage, given their problems of not acknowledging that they have a problem or their lack of motivation. The concern is that such individuals, if included in a group with clients at more advanced stages of readiness, might have a negative influence on those in the contemplation and action stages through their arguments that their alcohol and drug use is not a problem and that they do not need to change. Barrie (1991) also presents an overview of a five-session group based on the stages of change. The first two sessions, which deal with increasing commitment to change, are particularly appropriate for contemplators; the remaining sessions, which deal with developing general problem-solving skills and the prevention of relapse, are more appropriately targeted for those in the action or maintenance stages.

Despite these differences, Yu and Watkins (1996) and Barrie (1991) share a common view of the therapeutic tasks and goals for therapy groups at each stage of readiness. These approaches attempt to match the group interventions to the members' stages of change. Barrie (1991, p. 125), who was working primarily with heavy drinkers, lists the following as the objectives of such a group: "(1) to help identify problems related to drinking; (2) to maintain/enhance a commitment to change drinking behavior; (3) to teach methods of resolving drinking problems; (4) to monitor behavior; (5) to prevent return to problem drinking; (6) to help cope with a lapse." The following information, focusing on the general issues and approaches appropriate to groups at different stages of change, is derived from and integrates the work of Yu and Watkins (1996) and Barrie (1991).

Precontemplation Stage

Most precontemplators come into contact with treatment agencies through external influences such as legal, medical, employment, or social problems. They typically do not view themselves as having a problem with alcohol or drugs and thus are unlikely to consider a need for changing their behavior. They perceive the positive benefits of drinking or drug use and have not fully considered the negative consequences of their use. Given this position, a primary goal of a group dealing with precontemplators is to increase their awareness of their substance-related problems and move them toward the contemplation stage where they can begin to see a need for a change. Such groups, whether for only precontemplators or as the initial phase of a closed-cohort group, are often conducted as psychoeducational alcohol or drug information groups. Participants are provided information about alcohol and drugs, the negative consequences associated with them, and the potential advantages to changing their alcohol or drug use patterns. As Barrie (1991) indicates, the group setting offers clients an opportunity to reassess their situation and consider the extent to which substance use/abuse plays a part in their difficulties in a variety of life areas. A goal is to increase the individual's motivation for change by demonstrating the link between these difficulties or negative consequences and their alcohol or drug use.

Both Yu and Watkins (1996) and Barrie (1991) indicate that a group setting may be particularly helpful in dealing with participants' minimization of their problems. While group members may have difficulty in recognizing their own alcohol or drug use as problematic, they are often able to point out to others that many of the negative things happening in the person's life are the result of alcohol and drug use. Providing such feedback to a group member may also lead others (and themselves) to begin to explore their own use and the consequences resulting from it. Also, group members may be more receptive to input from other members—with whom they more closely identify—than from professional staff.

Yu and Watkins (1996) have noted that the therapist(s) doing groups with precontemplators should anticipate being the target of members' anger. The way in which the therapist deals with this anger is crucial. The motivational interviewing style would suggest "rolling with the resistance." By being objective, empathic, and nondefensive in response to the anger, the therapist models appropriate social skills and helps foster group cohesion, encourage movement in client self-assessment, and promote openness among the participants.

Contemplation Stage

Group members in the contemplation stage have begun to consider that the benefits of continued drinking or drug use may be outweighed by the negative consequences and that they may need to change. They are likely to be ambivalent and not yet fully committed to making such changes. A goal of therapy with contemplators is to increase their commitment to change. During this stage participants may be more receptive to information about alcohol and drugs, and, on the basis of increased awareness, they may begin to change their view of their alcohol and drug use, noting a shift in the relative weighting of the positive and negative consequences of their use. In addition to focusing on the individual's problem areas, the group should also provide information about available treatment resources and self-help groups that group members may find helpful in implementing change if they choose to do so.

It is likely that groups with contemplators will at some point begin to shift away from a more psychoeducational orientation toward a discussion format associated with more traditional process-oriented group therapy. The therapist(s) must guide the process to have members discuss their use patterns and resultant implications for current life problems. Such discussions enable all to share their own personal experiences in a way that both supports the individual's shifting attitudes and beliefs and provides feedback to others. Yu and Watkins (1996) note that it is important for the therapist to try to maximize the input from each group member in such discussions while assuming a less active role, serving to shape the discussion, correct misinformation, and reinforce group members' contributions and self-disclosure. They suggest that members may have a greater investment in the group process if the ratio of participant-to-therapist input is high.

Preparation Stage

Individuals in the preparation stage have resolved the decision-making challenges faced during contemplation. It appears that the move from contemplation into the preparation stage follows a shift in attitude about and perception of continued substance use. The negative consequences of substance use are now perceived as clearly outweighing the positive benefits of continued alcohol or drug use. This attitudinal shift appears to contribute to the now firm intention to implement behavioral changes. Clients have now firmly committed themselves to a change plan that they intend to implement in the very near future. Many may have already begun engaging in a variety of experiential and behavioral change processes.

As we discussed in Chapter 2, individuals in the preparation stage, in comparison with those in the precontemplation and contemplation stages, are more confident of their ability to change, already seeking out information about their problem and how it affects them and others, are stronger in their resolve to quit, are more likely to have sought out activities incompatible with substance use, are more likely to have rearranged their lives and environment to avoid high-risk situations, and are more likely to have developed personal and social networks that reward them for their decision to change. Thus, individuals in the preparation stage are high on dimensions related to both contemplation and action.

This bridging the gap between contemplation and action helps to determine a number of functions for the group. The major goal of the group in dealing with individuals in the preparation stage is to provide them with the support necessary to put an action plan into place and to follow through on their intention to change. Although the level of ambivalence has been reduced, the initial steps that are taken during the preparation stage are vulnerable to reversal until they have been solidified through trial and error. The group needs to develop techniques that further enhance commitment and that help to maintain change behavior. In order for the individual to move forward in the change process, as opposed to falling back, the individual's efforts must be reinforced, both by the group as well as through the development of self-reward contingencies. As these initial steps are reinforced, the level of self-efficacy will increase; the individual will increasingly feel more confident that he or she can deal with potential problems that might jeopardize the original commitment. In addition to providing a source of reinforcement for behavior change, the group can also raise concerns if they see the individual beginning to regress to a previous stage. The group can also help identify high-risk situations that may need to be avoided early in the change process, suggest other ways to cope with stress and strong negative emotions rather than by drinking or taking drugs, and develop contingency contracts that will serve as special reinforcers when treatment-appropriate behaviors are engaged in and negative sanctions if substance-related behaviors are engaged in.

Action Stage

The primary goals for therapy groups dealing with clients in the action stage are to reinforce their commitment to change and help them develop, implement, and test out skills necessary for them to change their alcohol and drug use. Barrie (1991) suggests that members should be taught general problem solving skills in which they identify and explore the parameters of the problem, brainstorm possible solutions, choose the most feasible alternative, put it into practice, evaluate its effectiveness, and make changes as needed to improve its outcome. Such problem–solving approaches, which are common elements in many cognitive-behavioral interventions with substance abusers (e.g., Monti et al., 1989; Kadden et al., 1992), can be generalized to any problem area. Group members, based on their experiences, can contribute to the brainstorming process by suggesting possible ways of dealing with a problem. In addition to merely discussing these alternatives, it is possible to have members role play them with other participants, with the therapist providing coaching and corrective feedback. The group may also serve as a source of support for the individual as he or she attempts to practice these new skills outside of the group session. Some group time should be set aside at the beginning of a session to review both successful and unsuccessful attempts at behavior change. Members who have been successful in their behavior change attempts serve as models for others who have been less successful.

The tasks for the therapist(s) in groups with clients in the action stage involve reinforcing the members' commitment to change, helping the group generate possible solutions to a member's problems, and reinforcing members' attempts at implementing the chosen strategies. In addition, the therapist(s) needs to guide group exploration of the possible barriers to change among clients who are having difficulties implementing their change strategies. Rather than being critical and confrontive, group interactions with less successful clients must be supportive, empathic, constructive, and reinforcing of the individual's self-efficacy and sense of optimism that he or she will be successful in the future.

Maintenance Stage

In the maintenance stage, group members continue to maintain successful behavioral changes until they become permanent, solidified, and relatively automatic. It is also during this period that members are successful in avoiding temptations to return to their previous alcohol or drug use patterns, anticipating situations in which a relapse could occur and preparing coping strategies to deal with it. Thus, group members are still involved in active problem-solving strategies and must remain vigilant of possible relapse situations. The function of the group in this case is to help the individual maintain a commitment to changing both substance use and one's lifestyle, maintain the therapeutic gains that have been made to date, remain aware of personally relevant relapse triggers, and support the individual's ongoing efforts (e.g., Donovan, 1998). Barrie (1991) notes that there is a shift in the group's focus away from drinking and drug use per se to the broader issues of lifestyle change. As such, groups with clients in the maintenance stage are more likely to be open-ended as opposed to time-limited.

Relapse

A major focus during the maintenance stage is on the development of relapse prevention skills. However, many group members may struggle during the maintenance stage and may experience a lapse or return to alcohol or drug use. A goal here is to support and reinforce the members' ongoing use of their successful coping strategies, minimize the likelihood of a lapse, and manage lapses that do occur so that they do not become more full-blown relapses. (We will discuss relapse in greater detail in Chapter 9.) Continuing care during the maintenance stage is often more effective in minimizing the harm associated with relapse than in preventing lapses from occurring (Donovan, 1998). An important aspect of this process is that group members have learned during the maintenance and relapse stages that relapse is common in the course of recovery, that it represents a component of the process of change and that many individuals who ultimately achieve success do not necessarily do so without temporary setbacks—rather, they may cycle through the stages of change several times before reaching maintenance. The hope is that the individual will not become so demoralized that he or she returns to the precontemplation stage but rather continues using the change strategies found most useful during the contemplation and action stages.

The therapy group plays a number of important roles during this stage. First, the group can be helpful in providing support for those individuals who are struggling and appear at particular risk for relapse during this time of increased vulnerability. It also serves as a source of support if a member does experience a lapse. Most individuals who experience a lapse feel angry at themselves, embarrassed, depressed, discouraged, and inclined to think of themselves as failures. The group must be willing to continue to work with and come to the aid of such individuals. Members who relapse, but have a positive attachment to the group, will be more likely to return to the group following a lapse. A group's history of providing comfort and aid to members who happen to relapse will also be a crucial factor. If those who relapse are spurned or confronted heavily by other group members, the end result may be a perception that the group "doesn't care" about the individual, is hostile and unsupportive, and increases the level of guilt experienced by the individual. It then becomes less likely that a member will want to return to the group if a lapse occurs. It is important for the group to remain objective, nonjudgmental, supportive, reflective, and empathic when dealing with a member who has lapsed. It is particularly important that the therapist(s) maintain this stance, model it for the group, and shape the discussion to en-gender this atmosphere. Also, having previously seen members who have lapsed return to the group, resume their therapy, reaffirm their commitment to change, examine the relapse situation to determine factors that may have served as triggers, develop plans to deal with these factors to solve similar problems in the future, take steps to make changes, and again achieve main-tenance provides a sense of hope and optimism to anyone who lapses.

"RESOLUTION-ENHANCING" EXERCISES
THAT CAN BE USED IN GROUP SETTINGS

The preceding discussion provided a general overview of the goals and objectives of therapy groups, based on a stages of change model. Barrie (1991) indicates that one of the overriding goals of such groups is to help clients to increase, solidify, and maintain their commitment to change and to learn and practice new skills to cope with problems as they arise and thus reduce the likelihood of relapse. Accomplishing this goal involves providing group members with opportunities for reviewing their sub-stance use, raising their awareness about its impact on themselves and others, increasing the perceptions of risks associated with use, and shifting the relative balance of perceived costs and benefits of continued use or changes in use. A number of "resolution-enhancing" exercises (Allsop & Saunders, 1991) may be useful in this process. These represent group ad-aptations of exercises that have been more commonly used in individual therapy approaches (Allsop & Saunders, 1991; Rosengren, Friese, Bren-nen, Donovan, & Sloan, 1996; Saunders, Wilkinson, & Allsop, 1991). These exercises can be performed during the group session by splitting members up into smaller working groups followed by general sharing and discussion, or they may be assigned as homework to complete be-tween sessions with the expectation that they will serve as a basis for dis-cussion in a subsequent session.

The Good and Less Good Things about Alcohol or Drug Use

The "good and less good things about alcohol or drug use" exercise (Allsop & Saunders, 1991; Saunders et al., 1991) provides an opportunity for the individual to evaluate the positive benefits and negative costs or

consequences associated with use. Saunders et al. (1991) suggest beginning with an exploration of the benefits of substance use as an empathic
approach that is likely to put the individual at ease. The client is asked to
list as many positive benefits that he or she associates with drinking or
drug use. This provides a backdrop against which the more negative costs
of use can be contrasted. Saunders et al. (1991) also note that such a review of the positive benefits provides the individual with a sense that
substance use may have certain rational aspects rather than being purely a
compulsive behavior outside of personal control. In the complementary
component of the exercise, the individual is next asked to list the more
negative aspects of substance use. Saunders et al. (1991) note that a
"softer," less confrontive approach of asking about the "not so good" or
"minuses" leads to less resistance than asking about the "bad things" associated with use.

Decisional Balance

The decisional balance exercise derives from the work of Janis and Mann
(1977), who viewed decision making as a rational process that involved
weighing the "pros," or perceived positive aspects, and "cons," or negative
aspects, of any behavior. This exercise can use the information derived
from the listing of good and less good aspects of substance use. However,
it also is useful to have the individual look concurrently at the pros and
cons of behavior change and/or treatment entry. The relative number
and strength of the perceived pros and cons can be compared to gain a
sense of the individual's current "leanings." The balance between the pros
and cons varies, depending on which stage of change the individual is in
(Prochaska, 1994; Prochaska et al., 1994). More positive benefits of
behavior change and more negative costs of continued substance use are
found in the action and maintenance stages, while more negative costs of
behavior change and more positive benefits of continued substance use
are found in the precontemplation stage.

Looking Back/Looking Forward

An important component of motivational interviewing approaches is to
attempt to raise the level of ambivalence the person experiences and
guide this ambivalence toward changing the individual's use patterns.
One method of doing this is to have the client look at the discrepancy

between his or her current behavior and personal goals or strongly held values. The Looking Back/Looking Forward exercise can be used to examine such discrepancies. The individual is asked to remember back to times before substance use became heavy and/or problematic and to compare how things were then in his or her life in contrast to how they are since a substance use problem emerged. The client is asked to respond to four questions:

1. Do you remember a time when things were going well for you? What has changed?
2. What were things like before you started drinking/using so heavily? What were you like back then?
3. What are the differences between the you of 10 years ago and the you of today?
4. How has your use of drugs/alcohol stopped you from moving forward?

In the complementary exercise, Looking Forward, the individual is asked to consider a changed future and try to imagine how things might be after quitting or cutting down on alcohol or drug use. The client is asked to answer five specific questions:

1. What are your hopes for the future?
2. How would you like things to turn out for you?
3. If you are frustrated in your life now, how would you like things to be different?
4. What are the options/choices for you now?
5. What would be the best results you could imagine if you make a change?

Exploring Goals

A related exercise, "Exploring Goals," asks individuals to consider those things in their lives that they feel are most important. These include such things as how the individual wants to be in the world, where he or she wants to go in life, the kinds of relationships with others that are highly valued, things he or she would like to do, and those things that are most highly valued. Individuals are asked to respond to four specific inquiries or requests:

1. Define your highest or most central values and goals (those things that are most near and dear to you).
2. List these values and goals in order, from most to least important.
3. What are some of the ways some of your behaviors get in the way, go against, or undermine your important goals and values?
4. How is your actual behavior different from what you tell people or what you tell yourself it is (are your actions different from the words)?

The "Miracle Question"

The "Miracle Question" exercise is adapted from the work of Berg and Miller (1992), who have developed solution-focused therapy as a brief intervention with substance abusers. The exercise is a method to help focus the individual's attention on his or her present adjustment and future goals. The "Miracle Question" is presented to the client as follows (Berg & Miller, 1992, p. 13):

> Suppose one night, while you are asleep, there is a miracle and the problem that brought you into therapy is solved. However, because you are asleep you don't know that the miracle has already happened. When you wake up in the morning, what will be different that will tell you that this miracle has taken place? . . . What else?

To assist in exploring the individual's projected future situation more fully, a number of additional questions may be asked:

1. Imagine a time in the future when the problem no longer exists—what will it be like for you?
2. How will your life be different?
3. Who will be the first to notice?
4. What will he or she do or say?
5. How will you respond?

The individual is asked to describe the perceived change in as vivid detail as possible, including any inner emotional responses generated by the image of the future. Berg and Miller (1992) note that the responses to this question lead to "miracle pictures" that are quite detailed and present potentially achievable goals. In addition to being useful in goal setting, this exercise also provides the individual with a sense of hope and optimism and also may contribute to an increased sense of self-efficacy.

SUMMARY

- Group therapy continues to be one of the most widely used approaches in substance abuse treatment. It has a number of advantages, as compared to other therapeutic measures, including the development of "curative factors" associated with the group process that may produce behavior change.

- A number of features of group therapy are thought to contribute to the process of behavioral change, including the realization that others share similar problems, aid in modeling appropriate behaviors, immediate peer feedback, and group support.

- A variety of logistical, practical, and conceptual issues need to be considered in developing a group approach. These include the use of an "open" versus "closed" group, homogeneous versus heterogeneous group composition, and the phase of recovery that the clients are in.

- It is important to develop within the group a culture that supports and encourages behavior change. Factors contributing to this culture are therapist style and group atmosphere.

- Therapeutic tasks and goals for treatment groups vary as a function of each stage of readiness, with group interventions geared toward members' stages of change. For example, a group dealing with precontemplators would focus on increasing their awareness of their substance-related problems and move them toward contemplation. The primary goals for groups dealing with clients in the action stage are to reinforce their commitment to change and help them develop and apply skills needed for changing substance use.

7

COUPLE TREATMENT AND FAMILY INVOLVEMENT

Substance abuse has often been described as a "family disease" (e.g., Goodwin & Warnock, 1991). This phrase has taken on a number of different meanings over time. One connotation suggests that alcohol and drug use disorders are familial in nature because of an apparent genetic predisposition toward substance abuse that runs within families and across generations (e.g., Goodwin & Warnock, 1991; Sheridan, 1995). The risk of developing alcoholism is an estimated seven times greater among first-degree relatives of an alcoholic than in appropriate comparison groups, with this risk being particularly high among the sons of alcoholic fathers (Pollock, Schneider, Gabrielli, & Goodwin, 1987; Merikangas, 1990). This apparent genetic predisposition has been more commonly found for alcohol problems than for other drugs of abuse (Bierut et al., 1998) and for the sons of alcoholics more than for their daughters (e.g., McGue, 1997; Muetzell, 1995).

A second meaning of "family disease" relates to the environmental context within which an individual is raised. While genetic and/or other biological factors are important in the etiology of alcohol and drug abuse, such factors alone cannot account for the risk of developing substance abuse (Steinhausen, 1995; McGue, 1997). Substance abuse generally develops within a family context, often one that includes alcohol and drug use and abuse by parents and siblings (Heath & Stanton, 1998). In addition to providing an inappropriate model for substance use, the families of substance abusers are often characterized by other problems, including a high degree of conflict, chaos, unpredictability, and inconsistent messages to children about their worth. There is a breakdown of traditional rituals and rules that are found in more stable family systems (Hawkins, 1997; Sher, 1997). Such environments are often associated with poor communications among family members (Murphy & O'Farrell, 1996, 1997), high levels of perceived stress (Kurtz, Gaudin, Howing, & Wodarski, 1993), domestic violence (Bennett, 1995; McGaha & Leoni, 1995), child abuse or neglect (Olsen, 1995), emotional and physical abuse (Famularo, Kinscherff, & Fenton, 1992; Kelleher, Chaffin, Hollenberg, & Fischer, 1994; Sheridan, 1995), and sexual abuse (Gil-Rivas, Fiorentine, Anglin, & Taylor, 1997). Children who emerge from such settings have increased risks for adjustment problems, including poor school performance, criminal involvement, depression, suicidality, and the development of substance abuse (Chassin, Curran, Hussong, & Colder, 1996; Ireland & Widom, 1994; Kurtz et al., 1993). Many individuals raised in such substance-abusing environments continue to experience emotional problems into their adulthood (Sher, 1997), including depression, anxiety, and posttraumatic stress disorder as well as substance abuse (Gil-Rivas et al., 1997).

There is clear evidence that substance abuse has a negative impact on the psychological and physical health of not only the substance abusers but also nonusing family members. Cook, Booth, Blow, Gosineni, and Bunn (1992) found that alcoholics with more serious dependence have a greater number of and more severe alcohol-related medical complications than less severely dependent individuals. Both the spouses and adult children of alcoholics have also been found to have higher levels of psychological symptomatology than comparison groups (Hinkin & Kahn, 1995). Holder and colleagues (Holder, Lennox, & Blose, 1992; Holder, 1998), in summarizing a large body of research, indicate that families of individuals with alcoholism have increased use of health care services. Roberts and Brent (1982), for instance, compared the health services utilization of members of intact nuclear families that included an alcoholic with those of matched controls from families not including an alcoholic. Members of the alcohol-involved family had significantly more physician visits and more medical diagnoses than did the comparison group. Of interest, this difference was found only for female family members; it may be that female spouses of alcoholic men are considerably more vulnerable to physical concerns or may see the family physician as a more acceptable resource than counseling or self-help support groups such as Al-Anon. The members of the alcohol-involved family tended to have a higher proportion of diagnoses of trauma and stress-related diseases, reflecting the difficult emotional environment of the family setting of substance abusers. This is consistent with the findings noted above concerning the negative consequences or correlates of substance abuse in the family.

Lack of cohesion within substance abusers' families is related to both the severity of the individual's and the family's psychological problems and to poorer prognosis of substance abuse treatment (Costantini, Wermuth, Sorensen, & Lyons, 1992). If the physical and psychological problems of family members as well as those of the substance abuser are not addressed, the effectiveness of substance abuse treatment may be compromised (Gil-Rivas et al., 1997; Stanton, 1997). In addition to possibly enhancing treatment efficacy and family functioning, substance abuse treatment, whether provided through formal treatment programs or voluntary involvement with Alcoholics Anonymous, Narcotics Anonymous, or Cocaine Anonymous, also appears to have a positive effect of lowering the posttreatment utilization of health services by both the substance abuser and family members (Lennox, Scott-Lennox, & Bohlig, 1993; Humphreys & Moos, 1996). There is also evidence that treatment of the substance abuser may have a preventive effect, serving to reduce the risk of developing mental health and substance abuse problems among the children (O'Farrell & Feehan, 1999).

Despite the negative consequences to the substance user and his or her family, a relatively small percentage of those with substance use problems enter into treatment (Marlatt, Tucker, Donovan, & Vuchinich, 1997). Bland, Newman, and Orn (1997) investigated treatment seeking by individuals in the general population who had been identified as having diagnosed emotional problems. While nearly half (47%) of the individuals with a major depressive episode sought help, only 16% of those with alcohol abuse or dependence sought help. Hingson, Mangione, Meyers, and Scotch (1982) found that only 21% of the individuals identified as having an alcohol problem considered seeking help when they first identified the problem, and only 15% actually did seek treatment. Of those who did not seek help, 84% said they did not believe their problem was serious and 96% believed they could handle it on their own. Over half acknowledged that they did not want to admit they needed help. In addition to the 15% who sought help initially, another 16% did so at a later time. Given that most substance abusers may not choose to seek treatment on their own, the family plays an important role in initiating the treatment-seeking process. Despite the problems that substance abusers generate for themselves and their families, they maintain fairly frequent and ongoing contact with parents, siblings, and significant others (Stanton, 1997). It is through this contact that family members may serve an important role, increasing the individual's awareness of the problem, facilitating treatment entry, and helping to encourage and support behavior change and maintain recovery.

READINESS TO CHANGE IN THE FAMILIES OF SUBSTANCE ABUSERS: A PARALLEL PROCESS

A family member's decision to take action and do something to care for themselves and/or the substance abuser is often a difficult one. The family, in its response to the substance abuser's behavior, is likely to go through stages of readiness to change that parallel those of the substance abuser. Early on there is often a tendency to minimize or deny that a substance abuse problem exists either for the individual or the family. Family members may be described during this early stage as being "codependent" or "enabling" since they appear, based on the absence of active steps to change the situation, to be supportive of the individual's continued substance abuse (e.g., DuPont & McGovern, 1996; Thomas, Yoshioka, & Ager, 1996; Whitfield, 1989). A television commercial for private treatment programs shows a family asking, "What do you mean, 'There's an elephant in the house.'?" The elephant, representing the alcohol or drug abuse problem of one of the family members, is standing in the middle of the living room, having nearly destroyed the entire house in full view of the family—yet, they are unable or unwilling to acknowledge a problem. Such a family is in the precontemplation stage.

Over time it is likely that members of the family begin to feel that something is wrong with both the substance abuser and the family. The negative consequences of the substance abuse, which persist and worsen, may clearly begin to be seen as outweighing the perceived benefits of maintaining the family and its dynamics as the status quo. A shift has taken place, with the family member, or the family as a whole, moving into the contemplation stage. There is continued evaluation of the situation. There is an evaluation of the family context, such as becoming aware that the children of the substance abuser have begun to have academic and disciplinary problems at school. There is also a more personal self-evaluation, in which the family member becomes increasingly aware that he or she is unhappy in the relationship with the substance abuser and more firmly determines that something must change in the family.

Moving from the contemplation to the preparation stage, family members have come to the point that they intend to do something in the near future and may have begun to take small steps toward change in the family system. They may seek out information about alcohol and drug abuse, attempting to raise their awareness of the impact of substance abuse on them, the family, and the substance abuser, experience emotional reactions to some substance-related event, and increase their awareness of alternatives to continued substance abuse within the family. One or more of the family members may become increasingly concerned and may begin to explore popular or professional literature, the local phone directories, Internet websites, substance abuse help-lines, as well as consulting friends, clergy, or health care professionals in an attempt to gain information to help them better understand substance use and dependence and to direct them toward possible treatment options.

At some point, the family member will attempt to take more notable steps to induce change in the substance abuser and the family system. The specific actions taken by the family member will depend on a number of factors, but might include leaving the relationship or getting support and help through counseling or Al-Anon participation for him- or herself as a concerned significant other in a substance-abusing relationship. This action might also include attempts to encourage the substance abuser's entrance into treatment and/or an active involvement in family/couple counseling to help the substance abuser, the relationship, or the family. It is important that the family as a whole, and its individual members, receive the support and encouragement necessary to take and maintain such steps; otherwise, there is a risk that, in response to the potentially painful process of change and the resistance from the substance abuser, the family will fall back (or "relapse") to its previous patterns of behavior.

Once having made the decision and taken steps to change, there appears to be a relatively consistent sequence of steps that the substance abuser, concerned significant others, and the family go through in the treatment process (O'Farrell, 1993b). These steps, which again parallel those found in the stages of change model, include initiating change and helping the family when the substance abuser is unwilling to seek help, stabilizing abstinence and relationships when the substance abuser seeks help, and maintaining long-term recovery and preventing relapse. Readers interested in more information related to many of the interventions associated with these stages are referred to O'Farrell (1993b) and Stanton (1997).

MOTIVATING BEHAVIOR CHANGE AND ENGAGING THE SUBSTANCE ABUSER IN TREATMENT

Many, if not most, substance abusers seek treatment in response to some form of external pressure from their spouses or significant others, physicians, employers, and/or the legal system. Hasin (1994) found such external social pressure to be highly related to help-seeking in a population sample of current and former drinkers, especially among those who had high levels of alcohol dependence. Krampen (1989) found a number of different reasons given for entry into alcoholism treatment. A subset of this sample was followed up for 1 year after completing treatment. One of the main reasons given by those who remained abstinent over the year was concern over the potential loss of one's marriage. However, drinking during the follow-up period was associated with already having had a spouse leave because of drinking. It may be possible to use such pressure and natural contingencies as a form of motivation to encourage treatment seeking by the substance abusers. In fact, Stanton (1997) has indicated that, next to legal coercion, pressure exerted by family and concerned significant others represents one of the most powerful routes to treatment entry and engagement.

A number of more specific interventions or approaches have been suggested for use in the motivation/engagement stage as family members begin to mobilize their energy and efforts. These approaches differ considerably in the degree of confrontation and coercion involved.

Johnson Institute Intervention

At the more coercive end of this continuum is what has become known as the Johnson Institute "intervention" (Faber & Keating-O'Connor,

1991; Liepman, 1993). Once a contact has been made by a concerned family member, the treatment professional makes an initial assessment of the substance abuse problem, the strengths, composition, and structure of the family and social network, and determination of who among this network should be involved in the intervention. These family members and other concerned individuals (e.g., coworkers, friends, physicians) are brought together initially to meet with a trained counselor, forming an intervention team. The team members are provided an orientation to the intervention process, are educated about substance use, are asked to formulate their concerns and feelings about the substance abuser and to determine what contingencies will be employed if the substance abuser does not comply with the intervention and continues to resist entering treatment.

Having practiced the delivery of their feedback, the intervention team members are brought together and the substance abuser is brought into their midst, often not knowing initially what is happening. Members then share their concerns and feelings with the individual, indicate that they hope the person will enter treatment, outline the consequences if the substance abuser refuses, and discuss the desired outcome of both the intervention and treatment. A referral to treatment is then made. In most cases arrangements have been made in advance with a treatment program so that, if the substance abuser agrees to follow through on the referral, he or she can be admitted directly with little loss in time and, presumably, in motivation. At a later date, members of the intervention team meet with the counselor to debrief their experiences and to lay out a change plan for the family to follow.

Liepman (1993) suggests that the Johnson Institute intervention is particularly useful in dealing with substance abusers who stubbornly resist entering treatment and who do not have any one person or institution that has sufficient authority or that can exert sufficient pressure to coerce the substance abuser into treatment. This approach is also more useful for those substance abusers who have a social network of individuals supportive of their recovery rather than those who have a limited social network or one that is composed of relatively superficial relationships.

To date there has been relatively little research evaluating the effectiveness of the Johnson Institute intervention. Gentilello et al. (1988) employed the Johnson Institute intervention with the families of 17 individuals who had been admitted into an acute care trauma center and were assessed to be alcoholic. All of the 17 patients who received this intervention shortly before their scheduled discharge from the trauma center accepted the referral and entered directly into an inpatient treatment program. Loneck, Garrett, and Banks (1996) found that alcoholics receiving the Johnson Institute intervention were more likely to enter treatment than were those who were referred through other means, both coercive and noncoercive. Those who entered treatment either through the Johnson Institute intervention or a coercive referral source (e.g., courts, legal pressure) were comparable with respect to treatment completion rates. It was subsequently found that those who received the Johnson Institute intervention had considerably higher relapse rates than those in other referral situations (Loneck, Garrett, & Banks, 1997). Clearly, while this approach appears to have potential benefits, it is in need of further evaluation (see the section on Community Reinforcement and Family Training later in this chapter for a discussion by Miller, Meyers, & Tonigan, 1999, on the results of a recent randomized clinical trial that included the Johnson Institute intervention as one of the treatment conditions).

A number of professional therapists and family members have chosen not to become involved in an intervention process (Faber & Keating-O'Connor, 1991; Miller et al., 1999). Liepman (1993) has discussed a number of ethical concerns that have been raised in response to the use of intervention procedures and that contribute to its not being a more widely used method of engaging individuals into treatment. The first has to do with issues of confidentiality about information that is revealed and discussed about the substance abuser, who has no say as to who will come to know of his or her substance-related problems. There is a related concern about the sense that the intervention, despite its presumably good intentions and focused goal of treatment entry, appears to be a "conspiracy" that may affect the substance abuser's personal freedom. Another concern has to do with the potential negative and harmful aftereffects of an intervention, either for the substance abuser or for his or her family (particularly if treatment is rejected). A third concern is that there may be a perceived, if not real, potential for conflict of interest on the part of the counselor conducting the intervention—in that the treatment program to which the person is referred often is affiliated with the program that employs the counselor.

ARISE Program

Given such concerns about the Johnson Institute intervention approach, a modified, less confrontive, but progressively more intensive approach has been developed. This approach—A Relational Intervention Sequence for Engagement (ARISE; Garrett, Landau-Stanton, Stanton, Stellato-Kabat, & Stellato-Kabat, 1997; Garrett et al., 1998)—is based on a number of underlying assumptions. These include the following: (1) involving the substance abuser in the process, where possible, provides a sense of respect for that person and encourages openness in the family system; (2) intervention is a process that falls along a continuum of increasing intensity of therapeutic and family involvement; (3) providing alternatives for the substance abuser to choose from reduces resistance; (4) the intensity of family and therapeutic interventions should be matched to the degree of resistance presented by the substance abuser; (5) there is a bond of caring between the family and substance abuser; (6) utilizing the strengths of a particular family or social network provides a sense of efficacy and the perception that it can overcome its problems; and (7) the family system benefits from and is strengthened by the intervention process even if the substance abuser does not enter treatment (Garrett et al., 1998).

The ARISE program is a graduated intervention that consists of three stages, each of which has greater family involvement, therapist direction, and possible coercion than the preceding stage. The first stage, described as an informal intervention without a therapist present, begins with a call by a concerned significant other to the treatment center seeking information about substance abuse and exploring treatment options. The substance abuser is resistant to the possibility of seeking treatment. Over the course of one or more phone sessions, in a manner similar to the Johnson Institute's intervention, the counselor assesses the nature of the abusers' alcohol or drug use, the circumstances surrounding it, and the social support network of the individual.

The network of concerned others plays an important role in motivating the substance abuser to seek treatment. The rationale is to involve these individuals in expressing their concerns to the substance abuser. The network group would be asked to attend at least an initial meeting at the clinic. They may be asked to attend 1 to 2 meetings per month over the first 3 months following the initial meeting as needed to facilitate the substance abuser's move toward treatment. Each meeting would consist of a number of components: eliciting a problem statement from each participant, reviewing efforts to engage the substance abuser, determining patterns of alliance among group members and with the substance abuser, discussing options to address the abuser's engagement problems, developing strategies to motivate engagement, and preparing to handle possible crises.

Up to this point, the effort on the counselor's part during the phone conversation(s) is to move the concerned significant other from the contemplation to the preparation or action stage, as well as mobilizing the social network in support of treatment. Commitments are made to have these individuals, as well as the substance abuser, invited to the clinic. The phone counseling also provides an opportunity for the concerned significant other to rehearse expressing his or her concerns.

While the counseling sessions over the phone can at times be sufficient to get the substance abuser to enter treatment, more often than not the process moves to the second stage, the informal intervention with a therapist present. Again, concerned others in the substance abuser's support network are invited to this meeting. This session (or several, if the need arises) is spent considering possible approaches that might be used to get the substance abuser into treatment. Emphasis is placed on expressing concern and caring for the individual, with the use of confrontation deemphasized. Again, an attempt is made to have the substance abuser attend this meeting. If, after repeated attempts, the substance abuser is still resistant and unwilling to seek treatment, plans are made to use the more traditional Johnson Institute-like intervention, which represents the third stage in the intervention sequence. Again, the use of confrontation is minimized and an attempt is made to maintain a more positive atmosphere. The ARISE model attempts to use the least coercive steps early in the intervention and then moves to those involving greater counselor and family efforts only if these lower-intensity steps do not succeed.

To date there has been limited evaluation of the ARISE program. A series of studies by Loneck and colleagues (Loneck et al., 1996; Loneck et al., 1997) have compared the Johnson Institute intervention with methods of facilitating treatment entry that differed in terms of the type of referral (either coerced or noncoerced) and the intensity of the process (unrehearsed and unsupervised). The unrehearsed and unsupervised interventions are similar in nature to the initial phases of the ARISE program. It was found that individuals in the Johnson Institute intervention were more likely to enter into outpatient treatment, equal in the rate of treatment completion, and higher in their rate of relapse than those in the other conditions. From these findings it may be inferred that interventions that fall at the lower end of the continuum of coercion are helpful and, among those who enter treatment, have similar completion and lower relapse rates than among individuals involved in the more coercive, staff-intensive, and more costly Johnson Institute intervention.

Unilateral Family Therapy

Attempting to provide support and increase the well being and functioning of individuals engaged in a relationship with a substance abuser is a primary goal of unilateral family therapy (Thomas & Santa, 1982; Thomas, Santa, Bronson, & Oyserman, 1987; Thomas & Ager, 1993). This approach, described by McCrady (1991) as promising but underutilized, attempts to influence the behavior of a resistant substance abuser indirectly by working directly with the concerned significant other. A primary goal is to increase the coping ability and overall functioning of the family by working directly with the concerned significant other. Changes made by the significant other may lead to modifications in the substance abuser's behavior, including the possibility of treatment entry.

Thomas and Ager (Yoshioka, Thomas, & Ager, 1992; Thomas & Ager, 1993) indicate that unilateral family therapy has three primary foci: (1) an individual focus that assists the concerned significant other by increasing coping skills and decreasing the emotional impact of substance abuse; (2) an interactional focus that assists the concerned significant other in mediating changes in family functioning by reducing nagging and other forms of negative communications, decreasing marital turmoil, and attempting to enhance the marital relationship; and (3) a focus on the significant other, attempting to help the individual develop more specific strategies to address the substance abuser's resistant behavior and facilitate treatment entry.

There are three main phases in unilateral family therapy with substance abusers (Thomas & Ager, 1993; Thomas, 1994). The first phase focuses primarily on the concerned other, preparing him or her to assume a rehabilitative role toward the substance abuser. The second phase focuses on developing specific strategies that can be used to influence the substance abuser to consider, seek out, and enter treatment. The final phase is a maintenance phase that focuses on continuing to work on the treatment and behavioral goals established by and for both the substance abuser and the concerned significant other.

Again, despite the apparent promise of unilateral family therapy to increase the coping and emotional functioning of the concerned significant other and enhance the likelihood of treatment entry by the substance abuser, there are insufficient empirical data to date to support its efficacy (Barber & Gilbertson, 1997).

Community Reinforcement and Family Training

An underlying assumption of behavioral approaches to family and couple's treatment of substance abusers is that the behavior of the substance abuser is governed by the principles of reinforcement. Therefore, shifts in the pattern of reinforcement and contingency management can be used to change the substance abuser's behavior. This principle is an integral component of what has been described as the Community Reinforcement Approach (CRA; Hunt & Azrin, 1973; Azrin, 1976). Sisson and Azrin (1993) indicate that, as they were implementing and evaluating a CRA program, they received a number of calls from concerned family members who were trying to enroll resistant substance abusers into treatment. Based upon the demand for services for dealing with such situations, they developed the Community Reinforcement and Family Training program (CRAFT; Meyers, Smith, & Miller, 1998).

The CRAFT program typically takes place over a number of sessions and has as its primary goals helping family members encourage the substance abuser to stop drinking and enter treatment. It also provides a focus on helping the concerned significant other learn how to take better care of himself or herself. The sessions focus on educating the concerned significant other about how to (1) reduce physical abuse and increase personal safety in the relationship; (2) encourage the goal of abstinence through contingencies that positively reinforce periods of prolonged abstinence and negative consequences for substance use that require the substance abuser to accept responsibility for the substance use and for making right the damage caused by this use; (3) encourage the substance abuser to seek professional treatment by identifying and attempting to capitalize on those moments when the abuser appears particularly motivated and potentially receptive to such a suggestion; and (4) empower the significant other to play an ongoing role in the treatment process through involvement in educational and therapy sessions.

If the training program is successful in getting the substance abuser to enter treatment, he or she is rapidly inducted into CRA (described more fully below). This will continue an active role of the concerned significant other in the treatment process through involvement in a family program used to provide ongoing monitoring of the use of disulfiram and in reciprocity marriage counseling. In addition to taking disulfiram, the substance abuser would be involved in social skills training, job club and vocational skills training as needed, the development of social, recreational, and leisure activities that are intrinsically rewarding to the individual and incompatible with substance use, and the development of skills to deal with the urges to drink or use drugs. Many of the contingencies that were developed in CRAFT prior to treatment continue during this active treatment phase. The goal is to reshape the substance abuser's pattern of behavior through the application of positive reinforcers and negative reinforcement.

Two recent randomized clinical trials have evaluated the effectiveness of CRAFT with alcoholics (Miller et al., 1999) and drug abusers (Kirby, Marlowe, Festinger, Garvey, & LaMonaca, 1999). Miller et al. (1999) compared three different types of significant other involvement. The first was a traditional Johnson Institute intervention, with concerned others developing an intervention plan and confronting the resistant alcoholic. The second was an approach that attempted to encourage involvement in Al-Anon, a self-help program for spouses and significant others in relationships with substance abusers (Cermak, 1989). Al-Anon provides support and change in self-perception of the significant other. There is no attempt to get the substance abuser into treatment; rather, there is the suggestion that one should detach from the substance abuser. The third approach was CRAFT, which combined elements of unilateral family therapy with those of CRA. Through the use of behavioral contracts and contingency management, the focus is on changing the pattern and contingencies of the substance abuser's social reinforcement, providing the concerned significant other with improved communication skills, and developing more effective coping and conflict resolution strategies. Each of these approaches was delivered as individual counseling sessions. The therapists in each condition used the particular approach as their primary mode of trying to get a resistant alcoholic into treatment; thus, they delivered therapies in which they believed and had considerable clinical experience. All the therapies were manual-guided.

The primary outcome of this study was the rate of entry into treatment by the alcoholic. Involvement of the significant other in the CRAFT therapy had the highest overall treatment entry rate (64%), compared to 30% for the Johnson Institute intervention, and 13% for the Al-Anon facilitation therapy. The vast majority (70%) of families involved in the Johnson Institute intervention chose not to follow through with the confrontation. However, completion of the confrontation was associated with a high rate of treatment entry (75%), versus a treatment entry rate of only 11% among those alcoholics whose families did not follow through with the intervention. A secondary outcome was the emotional adjustment of the concerned significant others in these three approaches. All three groups demonstrated significant reductions in their levels of depression, anxiety, anger, and family conflict and significant improvements of perceived family cohesion and relationship happiness. The improvements in these areas of function were comparable, with no significant differences across the three approaches.

Kirby et al. (1999) compared a unilateral community reinforcement training (CRT) approach with a 12-step self-help approach based on the principles of Nar-Anon. The primary outcomes of interest were attendance at and completion of the 14-session program, entry of the drug abuser into treatment, reductions of the drug abuser's drug use, and reduction of family problems. Secondary outcomes included mood states, self-esteem, social functioning of the significant other, and functioning of the family. At a 10-week posttreatment follow-up, the unilateral CRT was found to be significantly better than the self-help program on three of the four primary outcomes. Compared to significant others in the self-help condition, those in the CRT attended more sessions (8.6 weeks vs. 5.2 weeks of attendance), were more likely to complete the entire program (38.8% vs. 85.7% of scheduled sessions), and had higher rates of treatment entry by the drug abusers (17% vs. 64% treatment entry). Both groups demonstrated significant improvement, but did not differ from one another, on the reduction of drug use by the abusers, presenting problems, mood states, self-esteem, social function, or family function.

ACTION AND TAKING STEPS

The goal of the interventions described in the preceding section was to encourage and support the substance abuser's entry into treatment. Once there, the treatment may have varying degrees of spouse or family involvement, ranging from little involvement as a collateral informant to active and primary involvement in couple counseling. Regardless of the specific orientation or type of treatment, involving available family and significant others in the treatment and aftercare process appears to improve outcome. Peterson, Swindle, Phibbs, Recine, and Moos (1994), for example, found that involving patients' families or friends in the assessment and treatment planning process resulted in fewer readmissions in the year following discharge from inpatient care when compared to those who had no involvement by concerned significant others. Two therapeutic approaches to incorporate a spouse or significant other into the ongoing treatment are behavioral marital therapy and the Community Reinforcement Approach.

Behavioral Marital Therapy

As previously noted, substance abuse affects marital relationships in a variety of ways, including miscommunication, conflict, nagging, poor sexual relations, and domestic violence. Behavioral marital therapy (BMT), another promising but underutilized approach (McCrady, 1991), directly targets both the client's substance use and the marital relationship. This approach has been developed and evaluated by both O'Farrell (O'Farrell, 1989; O'Farrell & Cowles, 1989; O'Farrell, Cutter, Choquette, Floyd, & Bayog, 1992) and McCrady (McCrady et al., 1986; McCrady, Stout, Noel, Abram, & Fisher-Nelson, 1991). BMT can serve as an adjunct to or a component of more intensive substance abuse treatment or as a stand-alone outpatient intervention.

The initial step in BMT is a thorough behavioral assessment of the parameters of the client's drinking behavior; the environmental and interpersonal situations (particularly those in the family and marital relationship) that trigger and maintain drinking; the nature and stability of the marital relationship; current communication, conflict resolution, and problem solving abilities; the history and current risk of domestic violence; and other substance-related crises that may require immediate attention. The goal of the assessment is to target changes necessary to reduce or stop substance use and to improve the quality and satisfaction of the relationship. It also provides the context in which the couple can negotiate individual and couple goals that will be worked toward over the course of 10 to 15 sessions.

A number of specific behavioral interventions are used in BMT. Those focusing on reducing substance use directly might include goal setting for achieving either a reduction in hazardous drinking or abstinence, the development of behavioral contracts that define desired behaviors and the positive and negative consequences for either making or not making the desired changes in these targeted behaviors, the use of monitored disulfiram, the development of a hierarchy of both interpersonal and intrapersonal high-risk drinking or substance-using situations, and the development of specific coping responses for both the client and the spouse to address these situations. Interventions targeting the relationship might include communication, conflict resolution, and problem-solving skills training; the development of behavior change and contingency management contracts; and exercises to increase pleasing behaviors, positive interactions, and shared leisure and recreational activities (also see Rychtarik, 1990, for a discussion of alcohol-related coping skills for the spouses of alcoholics). The overall goal of these relationship-targeted interventions is to decrease the level of conflict and discord in the relationship, increase the positive feelings and goodwill between client and spouse, and strengthen the commitment both have for their relationship.

There is considerable empirical support for behavioral marital therapy. McCrady and colleagues (McCrady et al., 1986, 1991) compared three treatment conditions: minimal spouse involvement, alcohol-focused involvement, and alcohol-focused involvement plus BMT. Clients in all three groups showed a reduction in drinking and increased life satisfaction over a 6-month follow-up period. However, those who received BMT had a more rapid decrease in their drinking, had a longer period of time before relapsing, and maintained marital satisfaction better. A number of these initial gains persisted through an 18-month follow-up. While those who received BMT showed gradual improvement in the proportion of abstinent days, clients in the other two groups showed gradual deterioration in the proportion of abstinent days and light drinking days. Also, those who received BMT reported better marital satisfaction and well-being and had fewer marital separations. Similarly, Fals-Stewart, Birchler, and O'Farrell (1996), for example, compared individual outpatient treatment of substance abusers, with half of the clients randomized to receive BMT as an adjunct to their standard treatment. Those substance abusers who received BMT in conjunction with the individual counseling evidenced better overall outcomes compared to those receiving only individual counseling. In particular, these couples were separated less often and reported a greater degree of marital adjustment. Clients in this condition also reported fewer days of drug use, longer periods of abstinence, fewer drug-related arrests, and fewer drug-related hospitalizations through the 12-month follow-up period than those receiving individual-based treatment only. Not only were the outcomes better for clients in the BMT condition, but also the cost-effectiveness of BMT has been demonstrated (Fals-Stewart, O'Farrell, & Birchler, 1997). Provision of BMT resulted in a three times greater reduction in aggregate social costs than gained through individual therapy ($6,628 vs. $1,904). Also, BMT was more cost-effective than the individual behavior therapy, resulting in greater improvements in treatment outcome per unit of cost spent on treatment.

Community Reinforcement Approach

The Community Reinforcement Approach (CRA) is a comprehensive treatment that also has been identified by McCrady (1991) as promising but underutilized. The underlying principle of CRA is to provide the individual access to valued reinforcers contingent on his or her remaining alcohol- and drug-free; detected use of alcohol or drugs would lead to access to these potential reinforcers being removed and possibly replaced with aversive consequences. This contingency management takes place in the context of a number of other therapeutic components such as vocational job skills training, interpersonal and communications skills training, alcohol- and drug-free social club, and social support. As noted previously, the spouse or concerned significant other plays an integral role in the Community Reinforcement Approach, together with the substance abuser and counselor negotiating the behavioral contingencies, determining reinforcers, and establishing treatment contracts.

Contingency Management

An important component found in both CRA and BMT is the use of behavioral contracting and contingency management. In contingency management, an active attempt is made to change those environmental contingencies that may influence substance use behavior (Higgins, Tidey, & Stitzer, 1998). The goal is to decrease or stop alcohol or drug use and to increase behaviors that are incompatible with use. In particular, those contingencies that are found through a functional analysis to prompt as well as reinforce substance use are weakened by associating evidence of alcohol or drug use (e.g., positive blood alcohol concentration or drug-positive urine screen) with some form of negative consequence or punishment. Contingencies that prompt and reinforce behaviors that are incompatible with substance use and that promote abstinence are strengthened by associating them with positive reinforcers.

As an example, Silverman et al. (1998) evaluated the effects of a voucher program in the treatment of methadone-maintained opiate addicts with a history of cocaine use. Clients received vouchers that had monetary value contingent on providing cocaine-free urine samples. The value of the vouchers increased as the number of consecutive cocaine-free urine samples increased. Clients in the contingent voucher condition, compared to those who received vouchers on a noncontingent basis, reported both decreased craving for cocaine and significantly increased cocaine abstinence. It also appeared that the positive treatment effect was generalized beyond the primary focus on cocaine use, with clients in the contingent voucher condition also demonstrating an increased abstinence from opiates. Similar voucher systems have been effective in maintaining attendance of methadone clients in a job skills training program (Silverman, Chutuape, Bigelow, & Stitzer, 1996).

There is an increasing attempt to incorporate real-world contingencies into such programs (Higgins, 1999). Clearly, as noted above, programs can build contingencies such as take-home medication privileges into the structure of their programs. An example of a more real-life contingency management system is found in the work of Milby et al. (1996). Homeless substance abusers were enrolled in an intensive outpatient day treatment program. In addition, a group of these clients was also involved in a contingent work therapy and housing program. As long as the clients remained substance-free, they were able to remain in the job training/work program and remain in the therapeutic housing; if they were found to be drinking or using drugs, they were dropped from the housing and work settings. Clients involved in the abstinence-contingent program had fewer cocaine-positive urine samples, fewer days of drinking, fewer days of homelessness, and more days of employment during the follow-up period than did those in the standard treatment. Mark (1988) provides another example of such real-world contingencies. Approximately one-third of a group of substance abusers who were referred to treatment by a referral source (e.g., family, job, court, welfare, or child protective agencies) that had the ability to withhold anticipated rewards (e.g., welfare checks, return to job and a source of income, return to family) maintained continuous abstinence and treatment involvement over a 6-month period. In contrast, fewer than one-fifth of those substance abusers referred by noncoercive agents (e.g., self, friend, social agency, medical facility) met these same outcome criteria. Krampen (1989) has suggested the potential utility of other naturalistic contingencies. Threatened loss of job, spouse, or driver's license was positively related to treatment outcome among alcoholics. However, the prognosis was considerably less favorable in those clients who had already experienced a loss in one of those areas (e.g., the contingency no longer existed).

Behavioral Contracting

Higgins et al. (1998) note that often, but not necessarily always, written contracts can be used to help implement a contingency management program. The contract specifies clearly, often using the client's own words, the target behavior to be changed, the contingencies surrounding either making the desired behavior change or not, and the time frame in which the desired behavior change is to occur. The act of composing and signing a contract is a small but potentially important ritual signifying the client's commitment to the proposed change. In the contract, the client may include contingencies, especially rewards or positive incentives that reinforce target behaviors (e.g., attending treatment sessions, getting to 12-step meetings, avoiding stimuli associated with substance use). Goals should be clearly defined, divided into small steps that occur frequently, and revised as treatment progresses; contingencies should occur quickly after success or failure.

An example of a behavioral contract that is frequently used as a component of CRA or BMT is found in the descriptive report of O'Farrell and Bayog (1986). In working with couples having an alcoholic member, O'Farrell and Bayog developed a disulfiram (Antabuse) contract procedure. The procedure has three primary goals: (1) increase the alcoholic's compliance in taking disulfiram; (2) decrease the number of alcohol-related interactions and arguments between the alcoholic and spouse (which represent a source of stress and a potential relapse precipitant); and (3) increase the likelihood of the alcoholic maintaining abstinence. The alcoholic agrees to take the disulfiram daily while being observed by the spouse and to refill the disulfiram prescription before it expires. The spouse agrees to maintain a record on a calendar of the dates on which the alcoholic was observed taking the medication and to remind the alcoholic to refill the prescription before it expires. Together, the alcoholic and spouse agree not to discuss the alcoholic's past or possible future drinking (e.g., decrease nagging and drinking control efforts); to thank each other after the observed disulfiram use for being helpful toward one another and for doing something positive about the drinking problem; to contact the therapist if two consecutive days go by without observed use of the medication; and to agree on a time frame for the contract and on their willingness to discuss renewing or modifying the contract at that point in time.

The effectiveness of this disulfiram contracting procedure, as well as other behavioral contracting with substance abusers, has not been evaluated adequately. Most often, behavioral contracts and contingency management procedures are embedded in a more comprehensive treatment program. Contracts targeting goals supportive of recovery (e.g., improving vocational behavior, saving money, being prompt and regular for counseling and medication) are generally more likely to be achieved and may lead to better outcomes than those more directly related to substance use (e.g., clean urine samples) (Anker & Crowley, 1982; Magura, Casriel, Goldsmith, & Lipton, 1987; Magura, Casriel, Goldsmith, Strug, & Lipton, 1988; Iguchi, Belding, Morral, Lamb, & Husband, 1997). Iguchi et al. (1997), for instance, found that receiving vouchers contingent on completing objective, individually tailored goals related to one's overall treatment plan was more effective in reducing drug use than either a voucher system specifically targeting drug-free urine samples or the standard treatment without either of these contingency contracts added. The effectiveness of such contracts also seems to be linked to the severity of the consequences that might result from a broken contract (Magura et al., 1987).

MAINTENANCE OF BEHAVIOR CHANGE

While having a substance-abusing family member enter and complete treatment is an important step, it is equally important (possibly even more so) to maintain the therapeutic gains made during treatment once the individual has returned home. For instance, while Fals-Stewart et al. (1996) found considerable positive change in substance use and marital adjustment of clients who were involved with their spouse in BMT, some of the drug use and relationship adjustment differences began to dissipate over the course of a 12-month follow-up period. A component of the continuum of treatment targeting this phase of the recovery process is aftercare or continuing care (Donovan, 1998). In addition to involvement during treatment, involving available family and significant others in continuing care during the maintenance stage also appears to lead to improved outcomes. Two primary approaches of family involvement in continuing care are through behavioral contracts and relapse prevention approaches.

Behavioral Continuing Care Contracts

In addition to the behavioral contract to take and monitor disulfiram, described above, behavioral contracts have also been used to try to increase attendance at continuing care meetings following an initial more intensive treatment. A relatively easy to implement behavioral contracting procedure has been described by Ossip-Klein and Rychtarik (1993). It is negotiated as the client is approaching the transition from an intensive treatment (e.g., inpatient, day hospital, or intensive outpatient) to a less intensive continuing care. The counselor presents the client an appointment calendar for continuing care sessions and assists in negotiating an attendance contract between client and spouse. The contract involves the client's agreeing to post the appointment calendar in a prominent location at home, attend all scheduled aftercare sessions, and call to reschedule if an appointment must be missed. In exchange for adhering to these behaviors, the spouse agrees to provide a mutually negotiated incentive within 1 week of the appointment. The contract is then referred to at each subsequent continuing care session.

Evaluating the effectiveness of this procedure involved randomly assigning patients either to the behavioral contracting condition or to standard care during a 28-day inpatient program that routinely stressed the importance of continuing care attendance (Ahles, Schlundt, Prue, & Rychtarik, 1983; Ossip-Klein, Vanlandingham, Prue, & Rychtarik, 1984). Attendance was calculated as the number of patients attending each continuing care session at the scheduled or rescheduled day and time. In comparison to clients receiving standard care, clients in the contracting condition had significantly greater continuing care attendance, especially at the first continuing care session (72% vs. 36% for contracting and treatment as usual patients respectively), a greater likelihood of being abstinent at 3-, 6-, and 12-month follow-up points, greater rates of employment (46.7% vs. 13.3%) at the 1-year follow-up, and a greater likelihood to be considered treatment successes (77.8% vs. 38.9%, based on abstinence and reduced drinking).

Couple Relapse Prevention

Another avenue of family involvement during the maintenance stage is through relapse prevention programs that are integrated into couple counseling (McCrady, 1989; McCrady, 1993; O'Farrell, 1993a; O'Farrell, Choquette, Cutter, Brown, & McCourt, 1993; O'Farrell, Choquette, & Cutter, 1998). There are three main components of the relapse prevention process (O'Farrell, 1993a). The first is to help the substance user, the significant other, and their relationship to maintain the positive gains they had made during couple therapy. To this end, they are encouraged to continue with the contracted monitoring of disulfiram, relationship-enhancing shared activities, and attendance at self-help support groups such as AA and Al-Anon. The second is to deal with unresolved or emergent relationship problems utilizing therapist input and the communication, conflict resolution, and problem-solving skills gained in couple counseling. The third is to develop and try out a relapse prevention plan. This would include the identification of high-risk relapse situations and the early warning signs for relapse, and the development and practice of cognitive and behavioral coping skills to deal with these situations, and a specific plan of dealing with relapse if it occurs.

O'Farrell and colleagues (O'Farrell, 1993a; O'Farrell et al., 1993) have examined the benefit of adding a couple relapse prevention component as continuing care during the year following 5 months of weekly behavioral marital therapy. Participants were randomly assigned either to a condition that received no further treatment or to one involving 15 additional sessions of conjoint therapy focusing specifically on relapse prevention spread with decreasing frequency across a 1-year period. Both groups demonstrated significant improvements as a result of their participation in the initial behavioral marital therapy. However, those who received the subsequent conjoint relapse prevention sessions had more days abstinent, fewer drinking days, and improved relationships with spouses longer than those who received no further treatment beyond the behavioral marital therapy.

Self-Help Involvement

Dealing with the substance abuse of a family member is a stressful process. The concerned significant other and other family members may need ongoing support over and above that which they might receive from involvement in the substance abuser's treatment. This is one of the main roles of family-oriented self-help groups such as Al-Anon, Nar-Anon, and Alteen (Schulz & Chappel, 1998; Nowinski, 1999). These groups represent one of the most readily available and noncostly resources for family members; it is estimated that there are over 15,000 Al-Anon groups in the United States and Canada (Schulz & Chappel, 1998), which are based generally on the 12 steps and 12 traditions of Alcoholics Anonymous.

A major tenet of these self-help/mutual-support groups is that, even if the substance abuser continues to drink or use drugs, family members are able to get help through their involvement. Schultz and Chappel (1998) observe that two primary ideas are conveyed and reinforced in these groups. The first is that alcoholism or drug dependence is a disease and that the substance abuser is responsible for his or her behavior and recovery, rather than the concerned significant other. There is an emphasis on detachment from and letting go of the substance abuser, not being involved as an enabler of continued use. It is important to allow substance abusers to experience the natural consequences of their substance use. Group members provide support to the significant other as he or she tries to accomplish this difficult task. The second tenet is that the particular program is for the concerned significant other, not the substance abuser. The significant other has an opportunity and obligation to focus on his or her own emotional needs and self-esteem.

The studies by Miller et al. (1999) and Kirby et al. (1999) found that concerned significant others' involvement in 12-step self-help facilitation was less successful than CRAFT in getting resistant alcoholic and drug abusers to enter treatment. However, participants in these mutual-help groups demonstrated a considerable change in a number of areas of psychosocial functioning consistent with the goal of working on one's own needs. These studies found significant reductions in levels of depression, anger, anxiety, family conflict, and other presenting problems; significant improvements were also noted in family cohesion and function, and relationship happiness. The significant others in the mutual-help groups did not differ from those in the CRAFT with respect to these improvements.

SUMMARY

• Substance abuse is a family disorder, due to both the genetic predisposition toward developing substance abuse problems among family members and to the negative impact on the family, its function, and its members.

• Substance abuse treatment that includes family members or significant others is effective in reducing drinking or drug use, decreasing psychological and physical problems among family members, reducing health care utilization, and improving personal and familial functioning.

• The family and its members go through a series of stages in their attempt to deal with a family member having a substance abuse problem that parallel those through which substance abusers move in their process of change.

• Having come to the point of action, the family then must work to motivate the substance abuser to enter treatment.

• A number of interventions meant to encourage treatment entry have been used and evaluated. These range along a continuum of coercion from the Johnson Institute intervention through the ARISE program to unilateral family therapy and the Community Reinforcement and Family Training (CRAFT) program. A large number of families never come to the point of implementing the Johnson Institute intervention, but when this approach is used it appears successful in facilitating treatment entry. There is limited research evaluating the ARISE program. The CRAFT program is quite successful in getting resistant substance abusers to enter treatment and to change their behavior.

• Family involvement in the active phase of treatment appears to increase outcome success as well as family functioning.

• Both behavioral marital therapy (BMT) and the Community Reinforcement Approach (CRA) are effective treatments. Contingency management and behavioral contracting, components of both BMT and CRA, have demonstrated empirical support.

• Continued family involvement during the maintenance stage contributes further improvement over and above that achieved during the active intervention stage.

• Couple relapse prevention appears to be an effective component of BMT, leading to decreased substance use and improved relationship function. It is also a very cost-effective intervention.

• Mutual-support groups such as Al-Anon and Nar-Anon, which

are based on the 12 steps and 12 traditions of Alcoholics Anonymous, represent a readily available source of support for family members who are dealing with a substance abuser. While not being particularly effective in getting substance abusers into treatment, involvement in these groups appears to lead to positive benefits such as reduced anger, depression, and anxiety and increased self-esteem among those who attend.

• Given the positive effects of family involvement, treatment programs should attempt to include family members whenever possible.

8

POPULATIONS WITH SPECIAL NEEDS

Substance abusers represent a heterogeneous group of individuals who vary across a number of dimensions. These individuals may differ with respect to their demographic characteristics, presenting problems, motivations for seeking treatment, perceived barriers that delay or prevent their seeking and entering treatment, and needs to be addressed in treatment (e.g., Cunningham, Sobell, Sobell, Argawal, & Toneatto, 1993; Allen, 1994; Cunningham, Sobell, Sobell, & Gaskin, 1994; Siegal et al., 1995; Cunningham, Sobell, Gavin, Sobell, & Breslin, 1997). Many of these subgroups are also commonly underrepresented in and underserved by the substance abuse treatment system (Wilsnack, 1991). This view is consistent with an early definition of populations with special needs as populations or groups sharing common social, psychological, or legal characteristics that have encountered barriers in obtaining appropriate treatment (Diesenhaus, 1982; Institute of Medicine, 1990). Among the many possible populations with special needs, important subtypes that have relatively unique concerns and may require targeted interventions include women, minority ethnic groups, age groups (adolescent and elderly), and those with comorbid psychiatric disorders in addition to their substance abuse or dependence. For example, younger substance abusers do not find traditional, hospital-based treatment services attractive; it also appears to be difficult to attract women and minority substance abusers to such traditional treatment programs (Hartnoll, 1992). The constraints that make treatment entry difficult may be cultural, financial, and/or programmatic in nature.

Given the apparent difficulties in engaging and retaining such subgroups in treatment, the individual's stage of readiness to change may need to be taken into account and stage-targeted motivationally oriented interventions employed. Such approaches need to take individual difference, environmental, and cultural factors into account (Hartnoll, 1992). The purpose of this chapter is to provide a brief overview of a variety of clinical issues related to the stages of readiness to change in two such populations with special needs, namely, women and dual-disordered clients. We chose these two because they represent exemplars of populations with special needs and have received attention from the stages of change perspective.

WOMEN SUBSTANCE ABUSERS

The majority of research conducted in the area of substance abuse has been based largely on studies with men, raising concern that this information may not generalize to women. Recently, women have become the focus of increased attention in clinical research and practice (Schmidt & Weisner, 1995; also see reviews by Thom, 1987; Baily, 1990; Oppenheimer, 1991; Wilsnack, 1991; Smith, 1992; McCrady & Raytek, 1993; and Schober & Annis, 1996, for more thorough discussion of gender issues). Despite this increased attention, women are still often underrepresented and underserved in substance abuse treatment (Ramlow, White, Watson, & Leukefeld, 1997). As an example, while women represent approximately a third of problem drinkers in the general population, they represent only 20-25% of those who are treated annually in substance abuse programs. A survey conducted in the late 1980s found that about 25% of treatment programs sampled in a national survey provided specialized treatment for women (Wilsnack, 1991).

Reasons for Substance Use

Men and women substance abusers have been compared on a number of dimensions that may bear on the unique needs of women in treatment.

One area of difference is in the apparent reasons for drinking and using drugs. Men and women report different reasons for maintaining the use of the substances. In comparison to men, women have been found to misuse alcohol in response to stresses related to current circumstances or life events. This may be even truer for middle-aged women since a number of significant life events occur during midlife (e.g., divorce, bereavement, departure of children from home) (Allan & Cooke, 1985). Women also have a significantly higher prevalence of comorbid psychiatric disorders, such as depression and anxiety, than do men, and these disorders typically predate the onset of substance abuse problems (Brady & Randall, 1999). Consistent with this, Annis and Graham (1995) found that women were more likely to report heavy drinking in response to negative emotional states and interpersonal conflict with others than were men. Within this context, alcohol and drug use may be relied on more heavily to self-medicate mood disturbances among women than among men.

Consequences of Use

Negative consequences associated with substance abuse are different for men and women. This is especially true for what has been called the "telescoping phenomenon" (Brady & Randall, 1999). In comparison to men, women have been found to start drinking, get drunk regularly, experience their first drinking problems, and exhibit loss of control over their drinking at later average ages than men (Randall et al., 1999). Despite this later involvement in drinking, women have been found to progress faster than men between first getting drunk regularly and experiencing their first drinking problems and between first loss of drinking control and onset of worst drinking problems. Women also exhibited shorter average progression times between first getting drunk regularly and first seeking treatment, as well as entering treatment earlier in the course of their substance use problem than men (Piazza, Vrbka, & Yeager, 1989; Brady & Randall, 1999; Randall et al., 1999). However, this result has not been found consistently (Schuckit, Anthenelli, Bucholz, Hesselbrock, & Tipp, 1995). Despite apparent differences in the progression of alcohol- or drug-related problems, the sequence of their occurrence appears to be comparable across men and women (Schuckit et al., 1995; Schuckit, Daeppen, Tipp, Hesselbrock, & Bucholz, 1998).

Reasons for and Barriers to Treatment Seeking: From Contemplation to Action

It typically takes some time before a substance abuser seeks formal treatment for his or her disorder, often choosing to seek treatment only after experiencing significant negative consequences. The reasons that men and women give for seeking treatment appear to differ. While both report serious health problems as a major reason, men indicated that marital disruption was also important. Job loss, debts, legal problems, and homelessness were also important factors in the decision to seek treatment. Positive reasons, such as forming a new relationship, were also given (Thom, 1987). Thom found that substance abusers were more often seeking treatment in an attempt to alleviate problems other than their substance abuse. Few clients accepted referral primarily to change their drinking behavior. Women reported problems with children (fear of losing a child, recent loss of a child) significantly more often than men; men reported difficulties with aggression significantly more often than women. Among alcoholics who reported sobriety of one year or more, women more frequently cited relationships, while men more often noted their legal difficulties and status in the community as motivational influences on their decisions to become abstinent (Lutz, 1991).

Women experience a number of barriers that lead them to delay or not to seek treatment; these represent social factors, the characteristics of treatment facilities and the treatment process, and the personal characteristics and beliefs of the substance user (Jordan & Oei, 1989; Allen, 1994). One personal barrier noted by Wilsnack (1991) is *personal denial*, in which the individual minimizes the severity of her substance abuse problem. Even if there is an awareness of a developing problem, there is a reluctance to acknowledge it publicly and to seek treatment. Often this reluctance is related to fear of being *stigmatized* as a substance abuser (Schober & Annis, 1996). Marlatt and colleagues suggest that the fears about losing one's privacy, being labeled as an alcoholic or drug addict, and the stigmatizing effects of current treatments may be more powerful disincentives for women to seek treatment than denial of having a problem or structural factors such as treatment cost and accessibility (Marlatt et al., 1997).

Lack of social support for treatment, what Wilsnack (1991) has described as *family denial,* is another major factor in delaying treatment. The response to a woman's possibly entering treatment is often negative, even more so than for men. The spouses, relatives, and significant others often deny that the woman has an alcohol or drug problem and sometimes even actively oppose her seeking treatment. Beckman (Beckman, 1984a; Beckman & Amaro, 1986) found that nearly a quarter of the women in a treatment sample reported opposition from family or friends, as compared to only 2% of the men. As such, significant others' opposition to treatment is a key factor in outreach attempts to bring alcoholic women into treatment (Beckman, 1984a). Child custody and child-care issues also influence the decision about seeking treatment (Wilsnack, 1991). Women often have to find someone to care for their children while they undergo treatment. Also, women fear being perceived as an unfit mother and deprived of custody. Community leaders, social agency staff, and substance abuse treatment professionals agree that child-care accommodations at treatment programs are the most needed resource for women (Wilsnack, 1991).

In addition to these personal barriers, a number of factors related to the dominant treatment model and aspects of the treatment process have led women to be reluctant about entering treatment. A primary concern is that the most prevalent treatment model, which was developed to a large degree to address men, may not provide appropriate strategies to meet women's needs (Jordan & Oei, 1989; Ramlow et al., 1997). A major reason women do not enter treatment is that many treatment programs are not structured in ways that meet women's needs, nor do they provide gender-sensitive treatment services (Beckman, 1984b; Wilsnack, 1991; Nelson-Zlupko, Dore, Kauffman, & Kaltenbach, 1996). It may well be necessary to provide gender-specific support services (such as aftercare), child care, treatment for children, women's halfway houses, and all-female self-help groups to address many of the unique concerns of women substance abusers. There also needs to be sufficient financial support for women to be able to afford the services (Schober & Annis, 1996).

From Contemplation to Action

We can find points of intervention that respond to women's reasons for seeking substance abuse treatment, and the barriers to their doing so. First we need to focus on identification and motivation of treatment seeking in primary care settings. Often, and in particular for women, treatment entry is preceded by discussion of substance-related problems with a health care professional (Room, 1989; R. K. Price, Cottler, & Robins, 1991;

Bucholz, Homan, & Helzer, 1992; Marlatt et al., 1997). However, female problem drinkers and substance abusers are less likely than men to be identified in the primary care setting (Chang, Behr, Goetz, Hiley, & Bigby, 1997). It is necessary to utilize screening measures that have been developed and validated with women and are sensitive in the identification of substance use problems among women (Bradley, Boyd-Wickizer, Powell, & Burman, 1998). Thus, primary medical care settings may provide early contact points for problem identification and possible referral for substance abusers. Expanding the involvement of primary care medical providers may encourage appropriate help seeking and may reach substance abusers who otherwise would avoid traditional intensive treatments (Thom, 1987; Copeland & Hall, 1992; Marlatt et al., 1997). A similar identification and referral process should also be conducted in other medical and social service agencies that have ongoing contact with women, especially those settings (e.g., OBGYN clinic, pediatric services, emergency room, welfare office) having high rates of substance abusers in their clientele.

The more women perceive barriers associated with treatment, the less likely they are to enter treatment. Related to this, Beckman and Amaro (1986) found nearly half of the women, but less than 20% of the men, in a sample having entered into alcoholism treatment experienced one or more costs (e.g., problems with family, money, or friends) because of entering treatment. In order to increase the likelihood of treatment entry and retention, these barriers must be minimized, or there needs to be a way in which they can be addressed effectively.

Thom (1987) has noted that attendance by women at substance abuse programs often occurs despite the fact that they view other problems, not their substance abuse, as the main reason for seeking treatment and despite concerns that the program may not be particularly relevant to these other primary problems. Given that most clients experience such ambivalence about treatment even after entering it, and since this ambivalence may turn women away from treatment in the absence of services thought to be important and effective, it is also important to maintain or increase the motivation to stick with treatment. It is possible to use a number of techniques, such as a decisional balance in which the pros and cons of continued use and of treatment entry are weighed, as a means of increasing the motivation for and commitment to treatment (Brooke, Fudala, & Johnson, 1992; Cunningham et al., 1994; Prochaska, Johnson, & Lee, 1998; Donovan & Rosengren, 1999).

Another important approach to moving from contemplation to action is based on the family's reaction to the woman's substance use and the attempt to seek treatment. As we noted above, women encounter opposition to treatment from family and friends significantly more often than men (Beckman & Amaro, 1986). Beckman (1984a) indicated that overcoming the opposition of significant others to treatment is a critically important feature in outreach attempts to bring alcoholic women into treatment. So, involving the significant others in the treatment process, either as a member of a positive support network or more formally in couple or family therapy, is critical when resistance is encountered (see Chapter 7 for information about engaging significant others).

Female-Only versus Mixed-Gender Treatment: Action and Maintenance

Assuming women are able to overcome these barriers, take action, and seek treatment, a question remains whether women with substance abuse problems require different treatment approaches than men in order to be successful (Baily, 1990). The Institute of Medicine (1990), in discussing appropriate treatments for alcohol abuse, indicated that the evidence to date supports the contention that treatment programs that deal specifically with the problems that are more frequent concerns of women would lead to better outcomes. They also list those features of such gender-specific treatment that they feel would enhance treatment outcomes, including the following: "(1) child care, (2) assessments of psychiatric disorders and treatment for depression, when indicated, (3) methods of building self-esteem, perhaps through skills training, (4) support offered to and education of family and friends, (5) assessments of accompanying medical disorders, (6) availability of staff to work with families, and (7) teaching of coping skills for dealing with stress and other negative emotional states" (Institute of Medicine, 1990, p. 358). Also, in order to integrate the treatment necessary to address the broad range of presenting problems, case management can be used in conjunction with the primary intervention in order to enhance treatment outcomes for women in alcohol and drug treatment (Sullivan, 1994). However, the Institute of Medicine also indicated that further research is needed to determine the effectiveness of these treatment components for women (vs. men) and the characteristics of women for whom treatment is differentially effective.

Women who present to women-only programs differed from those seeking treatment in mixed-gender programs. Those in the women-only program were significantly more likely to have dependent children, be lesbian, have a maternal history for drug or alcohol problems, and have suffered sexual abuse in childhood (Copeland & Hall, 1992). In comparing the beliefs and perceptions of women in women-only versus those in mixed-gender programs, the women felt that these problems and related issues (e.g., such as low self-esteem, being victims of physical and sexual abuse, sexual orientation, sex-role conflict) could be met better in gender-specific rather than mixed-gender programs (Beckman, 1984a; Kauffman, Dore, & Nelson-Zlupko, 1995). Also, women who were able to have their children in treatment with them were found to have significantly better retention rates than those who were in treatment without their children (Szuster, Rich, Chung, & Bisconer, 1996).

Despite the strong advocacy for gender-specific women's programs, the results from studies evaluating treatment outcomes of such programs versus mixed-gender programs have been mixed. In a review of treatment outcome studies, Hodgins, el-Guebaly, and Addington (1997) indicated that men and women appear to benefit from different treatment approaches, with less structure required for women. Also, women appear to have a more restricted interpersonal style in comparison to men in mixed gender groups or gender-specific women's groups. On the other hand, Copeland, Hall, Didcott, and Biggs (1993) evaluated the outcomes of 80 women treated in a gender-specific women's program versus 80 women recruited from two mixed-gender programs. Both programs were based on the traditional disease model and the 12-step philosophy; however, the gender-specific program had only female staff and provided residential child care. Six months following treatment there were no significant differences in any measure of treatment outcome between the two treatment groups. Copeland interpreted the results as suggesting that simply providing women-only treatment and child care does not substantially improve treatment outcomes absent different treatment content.

Maintenance and Relapse

Treating women effectively also requires aftercare, relapse prevention, and gender-specific mutual-support groups (e.g., Beckman, 1984a; Wilsnack, 1991; Loneck, Garrett, & Banks, 1997). Just as men and women differed in the motivation for seeking treatment, there also appear to be differences in the reasons for or predictors of relapse following treatment

(Saunders, Baily, Phillips, & Allsop, 1993). Annis and Graham (1995), in their investigation of relapse precipitants among alcoholics, found that women were more frequently found among a group whose relapse risk was highest in response to negative emotional states. McKay, Rutherford, Cacciola, Kabasakalian-McKay, & Alterman (1996) had similar results in their study of precipitants of relapse among cocaine-dependent individuals. Women reported more unpleasant affect and interpersonal problems and fewer positive experiences before relapse than men, and their relapses were more likely to have an impulsive quality. Women reported more help seeking after initial use than did men (McKay et al., 1996). Consistent with this, women with long-term sobriety were significantly more likely than men to identify relationship issues as a primary motivation for their sobriety (Lutz, 1991). Based on these findings, women may need the greatest support, skill building, and relapse prevention training in dealing with negative emotional states, such as depression, anger deriving from interpersonal conflicts, loneliness, and low self-esteem.

Gillet et al. (1991), in a long-term follow-up of women who had received treatment, found that women who reported long periods of abstinence had been involved in a fellowship of recovering alcoholics. However, men and women appeared to respond differently to Alcoholics Anonymous, with women benefiting less than men (Tonigan & Hiller-Sturmhofel, 1994). This has led to the development of alternative self-help groups, such as Women for Sobriety (WFS; Kaskutas, 1996a), which represents a self-help option that is oriented toward positive thinking and behavior modification. The belief that behavior is dependent on one's thoughts serves as the underlying premise of WFS. This leads to a cognitive-behavioral approach in which members are taught that maintaining sobriety is based on believing that one can control negative thoughts and emotions and on how well one copes with these negative emotions. The goals of WFS include abstinence, improved self-esteem, and spiritual and emotional growth (Kaskutas, 1996a, 1996b). As is true of many self-help and mutual-support groups dealing with addictions, WFS is in need of further research into its therapeutic process and outcomes.

Summary

Although there has been increased sensitivity to the needs and issues that face women with substance abuse problems, this continues to be an understudied and underserved population. Women, representing one of a number of populations having unique needs, are confronted by multiple real and perceived barriers that make it difficult for them to seek out and remain in substance abuse treatment. These barriers are more likely to reduce the treatment seeking of women rather than men (Schober & Annis, 1996). To address the needs of women effectively, special efforts must be made to attract women into treatment settings and retain them (Sullivan, 1994). The interventions chosen should take into account the stage of readiness for change that a woman is in as she approaches treatment, engages in the treatment process, and maintains the gains made during treatment. Interventions need to be focused on the transitions from contemplation to preparation, from preparation to action, and from action to maintenance and relapse prevention.

While there is a continued need to look at factors that impede or help treatment entry, Brady and Randall (1999) have noted that many of the barriers confronting women who are seeking treatment are being addressed in many treatment settings, including family and couple therapy, as standard therapeutic interventions. It is hoped that such gender-sensitive treatment services will encourage more women to seek treatment, especially those who otherwise might not have done so (Copeland & Hall, 1992; Brady & Randall, 1999).

CLIENTS WITH COMORBID PSYCHIATRIC AND SUBSTANCE USE DISORDERS

Another population with special needs consists of those individuals who have concurrent psychiatric and substance use disorders. This group has become an increasingly large and difficult segment of the client caseload in both mental health and substance abuse treatment systems. While prevalence rates vary considerably across different combinations of psychiatric and substance use disorders, overall it is high when compared to those in the general population who do not have a psychiatric disorder (RachBeisel, Scott, & Dixon, 1999). Velasquez, Carbonari, and DiClemente (1999) note that the results of the National Comorbidity Survey indicate that over half the Americans who have a lifetime alcohol abuse or dependence diagnosis also have a lifetime diagnosis of some psychiatric disorder. Similarly, nearly 60% of those with a lifetime history of illicit drug abuse or dependence also have a lifetime diagnosis of a psychiatric disorder. Carey (1996) indicates that individuals with a mental disorder have a three times greater risk of having a substance use disorder than do those without a mental disorder. This rate is similar to that presented by McDuff and Muneses (1998), who also suggest that those with a substance use disorder, especially with drugs other than alcohol, are four to five times more likely to have a psychiatric disorder than those without a substance use disorder. Some subgroups, such as individuals with schizophrenia, have a particularly high rate of concurrent substance abuse (Carey, 1996; Addington, el-Guebaly, Duchak, & Hodgins, 1999; Bellack & DiClemente, 1999). Bellack and DiClemente (1999) note that the lifetime prevalence rate of substance abuse among persons with schizophrenia is close to 50%, and estimates of recent or current substance abuse among them range from 20% to 65%. These high rates of co-occurrence of substance abuse and psychiatric disorders have led Carey (1996) to suggest that such comorbidity may be the rule rather than the exception in some mental health treatment settings.

Nature of the Problem

The large number of individuals with dual disorders has had a tremendous impact on the treatment system. Salloum, Moss, and Daley (1991) note that clients with substance abuse disorders and schizophrenia are problematic from a clinical, economic, and health care systems perspective, placing a significant burden on the mental health delivery system through disability, social dysfunction, frequent rehospitalizations, and poor overall treatment compliance. Carey (1996) points out that, for some time, dual-disordered individuals were not treated in traditional substance abuse programs, and, if they were, they often failed to comply with treatment, left treatment prematurely, or had poor outcomes. As a result, the burden for treatment fell to the mental health system in some cases by default. In many cases, staff members were not trained to deal with these individuals—often referred to as "double trouble" since they not only have two disorders but also require at least double the effort to treat. Substance use or abuse tends to exacerbate these individuals' psychiatric illness; it also contributes to their poor compliance with medication and psychosocial therapies. As a result, the likelihood of psychiatric relapse is increased. Conversely, an increase in the experience and severity of psychiatric symptoms may lead to a resumption of drinking or drug use, with the individual attempting to decrease the experience of these symptoms through self-medication. The result of either of these scenarios is a poor treatment prognosis.

When compared to individuals with either a substance abuse or psychiatric disorder, those who have both concurrently tend to have more hospitalizations, more suicidal tendencies, poorer response to neuroleptic medications, less compliance with medication and psychotherapies, and a lower likelihood of receiving aftercare services (Carey, 1996). As an example, Stanislav, Sommi, and Watson (1992) found that 74% of individuals who had a comorbid psychiatric disorder and cocaine dependence who had been treated in a state psychiatric hospital were readmitted to the hospital within 1 year of their index treatment episode. Those with a dual diagnosis had a significantly higher rate of relapse compared to cocaine users without concurrent psychiatric diagnoses. Possible reasons for relapse incorporated both treatment system factors and interpersonal/social issues of the clients. These included lack of referral for substance abuse treatment, a lack of integrated treatment of psychiatric illness and substance abuse, lack of psychosocial support, and unresolved financial or job-related stressors. A similar pattern of poor treatment compliance and prognosis is also found in outpatient treatment settings (Carey, 1996).

McDuff and Muneses (1998) point out that it is important to have a full appreciation of the complex relationship between substance use and psychiatric disorders. As noted above, certain psychiatric diagnostic categories are more likely than others to be associated with a concurrent substance use disorder. However, they point out a number of other distinctions that need to be kept in mind. This relationship may take on one of a number of possible alternatives (Weiss & Collins, 1992; Lehman, Myers, Corty, & Thompson, 1994): (1) psychopathology as a risk factor for substance abuse; (2) nonpersistent psychopathology resulting from chronic intoxication; (3) persistent psychopathology resulting from chronic substance use; (4) substance abuse and psychopathology co-occurring and interacting to adversely affect the treatment responsiveness of each; and (5) substance abuse and psychopathology co-occurring but not interacting. Also, it is important to determine which of the two disorders is primary. Individuals may be primary substance abusers with psychopathology or they may have a primary psychiatric disorder with substance abuse (Lehman, Myers, Thompson, & Corty, 1993; Lehman, Myers, Corty, & Thompson, 1994). While both of these dually diagnosed groups have more life problems than individuals having a single disorder, the appropriate goals and approaches to these two subgroups among the dual-disordered population differ significantly (Lehman, Myers, Dixon, & Johnson, 1994; McDuff & Muneses, 1998).

Role of Substance Use

Another important consideration in dealing with dual-disordered clients is the role(s) played or the function(s) served by alcohol or drugs. A thorough behavioral assessment and functional analysis provide information about the functional utility of alcohol and drugs, the antecedents and consequences of use, and the "triggers" or high-risk situations that are most commonly associated with drinking or taking drugs (Stasiewicz, Carey, Bradizza, & Maisto, 1996). Bellack and DiClemente (1999) observe that a common assumption is that schizophrenics use substances to reduce their experience of psychotic symptoms and/or to alleviate the sedating side effects of neuroleptic medications. Drake, McLaughlin, Pepper, and Minkoff (1991) also indicate that an attempt at alleviating or self-medicating the symptoms of schizophrenia or the side effects of psychotropic medications represents one possible reason for use. They also suggest that attempts to develop an identity that is more acceptable and less stigmatizing than that of a "mental patient" (e.g., an "alcoholic" or "drug addict") and an attempt to encourage social interactions may be additional reasons for use.

However, the most common reasons typically given for use of alcohol and other drugs is to "get high" and to reduce negative affective states, including social anxiety and tension, dysphoria and depression, and boredom (Carey & Carey, 1995; Bellack & DiClemente, 1999). Consistent with this, Bradizza, Stasiewicz, and Carey (1998) found that clients with serious mental illnesses who had either a concurrent alcohol or drug use disorder both reported using substances most frequently when feeling anxiety or depressive symptoms (including helplessness, hopelessness, and worthlessness) rather than psychotic symptoms. Symptoms of hearing voices or experiencing hallucinations were among the least frequently endorsed reasons for using. Among those who abused alcohol, response to such negative emotional states was the most prominent trigger of drinking, while social pressure to use and wanting to share pleasant times with others were the most prominent reasons among those who abused drugs. These findings suggest that, as with substance abusers without a concurrent psychiatric disorder, alcohol and drug use may represent an attempt to cope with negative mood states in the absence of more appropriate and adaptive cognitive, behavioral, and emotional coping abilities.

Although based on a small sample and considered to be preliminary, the results of Bradizza et al. (1998) suggest the importance of behavioral treatment interventions such as coping skills training, stimulus control techniques, and relapse prevention. Those dual-disordered clients with an alcohol use disorder may benefit most from general social skills training and more specifically focused training in dealing with negative emotional states. Those with primarily a drug use disorder may benefit more from skills training that focuses on interpersonal issues, such as methods to deal with social pressures to use and other ways to interact with people without using drugs.

Treatment Considerations

Limitations in Traditional Substance Abuse Treatment

As we noted above, traditional substance abuse treatment does not appear to be particularly effective with individuals with dual disorders, for a number of reasons. First, individuals with major psychiatric disorders, with or without comorbid substance abuse, appear less able to deal with the high level of affect, interpersonal intensity, and confrontive styles often found in substance abuse programs (Bellack & DiClemente, 1999). Second, substance abuse programs often proceed at a fairly rapid, often lockstep, pace. Individuals with dual disorders appear to benefit more from a slower and more structured approach to treatment (McDuff & Muneses, 1998). Third, substance abuse programs often have fairly rigid rules and expectations for behavior, often using ultimatums as a means of forcing compliance; it appears that dual-disordered clients do better with a greater degree of flexibility in the treatment process (Smyth, 1996). One area in which this has become increasingly clear is the expectation of abstinence as a condition for continued involvement in treatment. This is often an expectation in many substance abuse programs. However, there is a concern that, while this represents a long-term goal, individuals with dual disorders have greater difficulty achieving and maintaining abstinence than substance abusers who do not have concurrent psychiatric disorders. Withholding necessary psychotherapeutic and pharmacological treatments from dual-disordered clients who are unable to become or remain abstinent may further worsen their condition.

Need for Specialized Programs

Based on these considerations, considerable discussion has occurred about the most productive methods to use to treat this population. A number of options have been suggested and implemented. Ries (1993, 1994) has reviewed the models of treatment that have been used in treating individuals with dual disorders. The first is *sequential* treatment. The individual is treated initially for one of the two disorders, typically the one representing the presenting problem, followed by subsequent treatment of the second disorder. The second is *parallel* treatment. The individual is receiving treatment concurrently but in two different clinics or treatment systems. These two approaches were the ones used during the earlier stages of dual-disorder treatment. A major problem is that these two approaches often left much of the responsibility for integrating and adapting to different and sometimes conflicting treatment models. The result was that many clients "dropped through the cracks," failing to make the transition between the two programs and never effectively engaging in the second treatment program. Also, there is a high degree of coordination necessary among the clinical staff of different programs to ensure that the client enters and complies with treatment in both systems. Also, in both the parallel and sequential models, dual-disordered clients received traditional substance abuse treatment, which, as noted above, does not appear to be the most appropriate and efficacious approach. Some of the concerns about coordination across programs and staff have been lessened by the increased use of case management services, which are felt to be critical for effective treatment of this population (Ries, 1994; Drake & Noordsy, 1997).

The difficulties experienced in both the sequential and parallel models have led to the development of specialized, integrated dual-disorder treatment programs. In the *integrated* model, individuals receive treatment for both disorders concurrently within a single treatment program. These programs have been established in both inpatient (e.g., Bradizza & Stasiewicz, 1997) and outpatient settings (e.g., Carey, 1996). While providing more coordinated care and demonstrating encouraging results (Drake, Mercer-McFadden, Mueser, McHugo, & Bond, 1998), the integrated approach is not without problems. One is that it is necessary to have staff who are knowledgeable about both psychiatric and substance use disorders and have the clinical skill to deal with this group. Smyth (1996) has noted another potential problem for the integrated approach. This approach has difficulty in dealing with clients having widely varying severity in either or both psychiatric and substance abuse in the same program. Many clients with dual disorders acknowledge only one (or neither) of the problems, resulting in their being at different stages of acceptance of and willingness/readiness to change each problem. Failure to accept one or the other disorder (or both) can be a formidable barrier to change (Smyth, 1996).

Carey (1996) has suggested that specialized treatments for dual-disordered individuals should incorporate a number of features that can be derived from more recent advances in substance abuse treatment. Each of these addresses one or more of the concerns noted in attempting to deal with dual-disordered individuals in more traditional substance abuse programs. The first is that the intensity of treatment should be matched to the severity of the disorder, both with respect to the psychiatric and substance use problems. This is true for treatment provided in both inpatient and outpatient settings (Kofoed, 1993). Second, these individuals vary in their readiness to change their behavior. Any model of treatment must then incorporate awareness of stages of change and include strategies to ready clients for active change. Third, motivational interviewing techniques can be used to enhance motivation to change addictive behaviors. Its reliance on supportive, nonconfrontational, and collaborative interventions is designed to minimize defensiveness and resistance to change and to increase self-efficacy. Fourth, a harm reduction approach is warranted. A basic assumption of harm reduction is that substance use falls along a continuum from abstinence to problematic use or abuse. While abstinence and a substance-free life represent long-term goals, any intermediate step in that direction, such as reducing the quantity and/or frequency of use, should be viewed positively and reinforced.

Stages of Treatment

A conceptual clinical model of dual-disorder treatment has incorporated a stage approach. Kofoed and colleagues (Osher & Kofoed, 1989; Kofoed, 1993; Kofoed, 1997) suggest at least four stages in the treatment process:

(1) engagement, (2) persuasion, (3) active treatment, and (4) relapse prevention. An important focus of this approach is its emphasis on the early phase of the treatment process. As Carey (1996) noted, the bulk of treatments developed for substance abusers focus on active change and relapse prevention. Greater consideration must be given to effective engagement techniques, clients' readiness for active treatment, and matching phases of intervention with phases of the clients' acceptance of his or her dual problems (Addington et al., 1999). As McDuff and Muneses (1998) state, "Persuading dually diagnosed patients to acknowledge that a problem exists and that treatment is warranted is challenging for even the most experienced clinician" (p. 41).

Focus on Engagement and Persuasion

Many dual-disordered individuals do not feel that they have a problem, instead appearing to be in "dual denial" (Smyth, 1996). They also might be what McDuff and Muneses (1998) describe as "reluctant" pre-contemplators, in which the deficits associated with their psychiatric disorder keep them from being fully aware of or understanding the impact of their problems, and it is this lack of knowledge that keeps them from wanting to change their behaviors. Others may admit to having psychiatric problems but not substance use problems. They may rationalize their substance use, suggesting that it is just their way of trying to cope with their "real" problem (McDuff & Muneses, 1998). Others may suggest that they are already doing something about their problem(s) while there does not appear to be any effort noticeable from an outside perspective. Addington et al. (1999) interviewed schizophrenics involved in outpatient treatment who had concurrent alcohol or drug use disorders. The clients also completed a measure of stages of change. It was found that there was little agreement between the stages of change based on the clinical interview and clients' self-reports. In most cases, the individuals rated themselves as being in a stage of action, while they were rated by the clinician as actually being in either precontemplation or contemplation.

Clearly, to be most successful, both the psychiatric and substance abuse problems must be addressed. A prerequisite for this is that the individual must have some awareness of having problems and some degree of willingness to accept the need for change and for treatment (Salloum et al., 1998). A number of authors have recommended the use of decisional balance techniques to help increase the level of problem awareness. However, there have been concerns expressed (e.g., Bellack & DiClemente, 1999) that deficits in self-awareness, abstract reasoning, judgment, and problem solving that accompany such severe psychiatric disorders as schizophrenia would inevitably make it difficult to evaluate the pros and cons of continued substance use. However, this does not seem to be as problematic as anticipated. Carey, Purnine, Maisto, Carey, and Barnes (1999) found that schizophrenics with concurrent substance use disorders were able to engage in the decisional balance process and generate a range of pros and cons of both continued use and quitting use.

Velasquez et al. (1999) have hypothesized that the pros of drinking would be positively related to psychiatric severity among dual-disordered clients with an alcohol use disorder; those with higher distress would see more benefits from drinking and would endorse more pros than those with less severe psychiatric problems. Conversely, those with greater severity would endorse fewer cons, or negative consequences of drinking. However, those clients who had more severe psychiatric and drinking problems were much more aware of the cons of drinking than were those with lower problem severity. Stasiewicz, Bradizza, and Maisto (1997) found that negative life events and weighing the pros and cons of drinking were most often associated with entry into treatment among a group of individuals with severe psychiatric disorders and comorbid alcohol use disorders than were positive life events and advice or warnings from others.

Kofoed (1997) noted that another important process in attempting to engage dual-disordered individuals in treatment is instillation of hope. This is similar to the goal of increasing self-efficacy within a stage of change and motivational enhancement model. He notes that many individuals with severe psychiatric disorders and substance abuse are characterized by extreme demoralization and a sense of futility derived from their past experiences, which often include prior treatment failures. Further, he suggests that much of what is viewed as treatment refusal or lack of readiness for treatment stems from this demoralization. The task of the clinician is to provide a sense of optimism that treatment can be effective and that there are rewarding alternatives to substance use. Further, from the standpoint of enhancing self-efficacy, it is important to instill a belief not only that change is possible but also that the individual is capable of making positive changes. In addition to addressing these issues in therapeutic sessions, McDuff and Muneses (1998) also suggest matching the precontemplator with an empathic recovering individual whose experience indicates that others with similar problems have been successful through involvement in treatment.

Active Treatment

Once the individual has become engaged enough to consider and possibly begin treatment, the action phase has been entered. Carey (1996) has outlined the main components of a dual-disorders treatment program that would fit into a mental health center system with clients assigned primary case managers. These include (1) establishing a working therapeutic alliance between client and therapist, (2) conducting a decisional balance, evaluating the cost-benefit ratio of continued substance use, (3) individualizing goals for changes in substance use, with harm reduction through decreased quantity and frequency of use being acceptable, (4) building an environment and lifestyle supportive of abstinence, and (5) anticipating and coping with crises.

Bellack and DiClemente (1999) have also described an outpatient treatment program for schizophrenics with comorbid substance use disorders. It was designed to take into account the unique deficits in motivation, cognitive function, and social skills associated with schizophrenia. It consists of four modules that are introduced sequentially: (1) social skills and problem solving as a means of increasing clients' development of social contacts with others who are not using drugs and of becoming better able at refusing social pressure to use substances; (2) education about reasons for substance use, including habits, triggers, craving, and the particular dangers of substance abuse for those with schizophrenia; (3) motivational interviewing, goal setting for decreasing substance use, and development of contingency contracts for negative drug urine tests, which provides an incentive/motivation for not using; and (4) training in behavioral skills for coping with urges and high-risk situations, and relapse prevention skills.

This treatment is delivered in a small-group format with six to eight clients. Group sessions are 90 minutes long, with two sessions per week over approximately a 6-month treatment period. This approach relies heavily on instruction, modeling, role playing, feedback and positive reinforcement, and homework. It initially focuses on increasing self-efficacy through achieving success in learning, and using skills both within the group as well as outside treatment. A decisional balance procedure is also included in the treatment. However, rather than attempting to consider a large number of consequences or ones that are somewhat global in nature, the focus instead is on one or two specific negative consequences that have a strong impact on the person and his or her symptoms and can thus serve as a prompt for change. The treatment also incorporates a harm reduction orientation, with successive approximations toward abstinence being reinforced.

Transitions in Treatment

While there is a trend toward more integrated dual-disorders treatment programs, many settings are not able to develop or implement such an approach. These often continue to rely on the sequential or parallel models of treatment, which require clients to move from one program to another. Also, given the chronicity and severity of many types of psychiatric and substance use disorders, clients often need various levels of treatment during the course of recovery; these may be delivered by different staff in different treatment settings (e.g., inpatient, day hospital, outpatient) (Kofoed, 1993; Daley & Salloum, 1999). As noted above, a risk in such circumstances is that clients will "fall through the cracks" in the transitions between programs or levels of care.

Two studies have recently investigated the impact of motivational interviews with dual-disordered clients as they transitioned from inpatient to outpatient settings. Daley and Zuckoff (1998) evaluated the utility of a single motivational therapy session prior to hospital discharge aimed at increasing compliance with outpatient treatment. The rates of attendance at the first postdischarge outpatient appointment were compared for patients prior to and following the introduction of the motivational session. The attendance rate at the initial outpatient appointment increased from 35% prior to the introduction of the motivational session to 67% afterward. Swanson, Pantalon, and Cohen (1999) also looked at the effect of motivational enhancement on the postdischarge outpatient session adherence among dually diagnosed inpatients. Dual-disordered patients were randomly assigned to standard inpatient care, which included pharmacotherapy, individual and group psychotherapy, activity therapy, milieu therapy, and discharge planning, or to standard care plus a motivational enhancement session. Motivational enhancement consisted of a 15-minute feedback on the results of a motivational assessment early in the hospitalization and a 1-hour motivational interview before discharge. The clinicians used the principles and techniques of motivational interviewing, including reflective listening, discussion of treatment obstacles, and elicitation of motivational self-statements. Those dual-disordered patients who received the motivational interview were significantly more likely to attend their initial outpatient appointment (42%) than were those who received standard care without the motivational session (16%). While the results of these studies are encouraging in showing that brief motivational interventions can increase attendance and reduce attrition during transitions in treatment, the absolute values of clients attending indicates that there is considerable room for improvement.

SUMMARY

• The substance-abusing population is heterogeneous, composed of a number of clinically meaningful subgroups of individuals having special needs.

• It is important to be aware of the unique characteristics of clients, the needs that they present, and the barriers that may interfere with treatment and behavior change.

• Evidence suggests that outcomes are improved if the treatment services provided meet the specific needs of the client.

• A major area where special-needs clients have difficulty is in the process of treatment seeking and engagement.

• The stages of change model provides a heuristic model through which to understand the difficulties in treatment engagement of clients with special needs.

• An important element of engagement is the instillation of hope, the belief that treatment is effective and that the client can change. This contributes to increased self-efficacy.

• Decisional balance procedures appear to be effective in helping to persuade clients that they have a problem(s) and that change would be beneficial.

• A harm reduction philosophy, in which decreases in quantity and frequency of substance use are reinforced and seen as intermediate steps toward a longer-term goal of abstinence, is more likely to lead to treatment engagement than strict abstinence-only philosophies in certain subgroups, such as those with dual disorders.

- Transitions from one program to another or from one level of care to another within a treatment system result in high attrition rates. Motivational interviewing appears to be effective in reducing attrition and in increasing treatment attendance.

9

RELAPSE

Relapse is an old and still challenging problem in the addictive behaviors. In the most general sense, relapse refers to a return to a problematic behavior. The high rates at which individuals return to substance use after stopping for any particular period of time supports the belief among many counselors and clients that, tough as it may be for a client to quit use of a substance, "staying quit" is even tougher. In this regard, Washton (1988) noted that "traditionally, relapse has been the nemesis of addiction treatment for all types of chemical dependency problems, including alcohol, heroin, and other drugs" (p. 34). Similarly, Rounsaville (1986) has argued that "relapse and relapse prevention define the major clinical problems to be faced by clinicians and researchers who do work with substance abusers" (p. 172).

Although precise figures on the prevalence of relapse are not available, there are strong indications that relapses are anything but uncommon. Hunt, Barnett, and Branch (1971) summarized relapse rates for a variety of substances. As shown in Figure 9.1, individuals treated for heroin, smoking, and alcohol addiction exhibit high rates of relapse. Indeed, approximately two-thirds of these clients had relapsed within the initial 3 months following the conclusion of treatment.

While the data summarized by Hunt et al. (1971) clearly highlight the prevalence of relapse events, keep in mind that relapse for purposes of

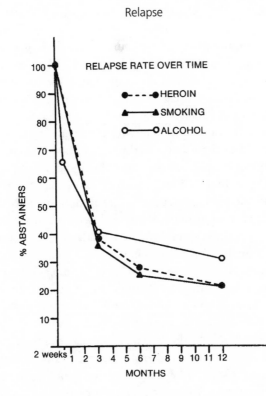

FIGURE 9.1. Relapse rates over time for clients treated for heroin, smoking, and alcohol addiction. From Hunt, Barnett, and Branch (1971, p. 455). Copyright 1971 by the Clinical Psychology Publishing Co., Inc. Reprinted by permission of John Wiley & Sons, Inc.

the Hunt et al. (1971) study was defined as any return to the use of the respective substances, without reference to the amount of the substance used or the duration of use. As such, persons who took one drink (in the alcohol category) and then returned to abstinence would be viewed no differently than persons who drank heavily and over an extended period of time. Clearly, use of different definitions of relapse (a single use of a drug versus 5 days of continuous use, as an example) affects the rate of relapse indicated. The case of relapse among alcoholics serves as a useful illustration. When defining relapse as a return to pretreatment levels of drinking, Armor, Polich, and Stambul (1978) found a relapse rate of around 50% over a 12-month posttreatment follow-up period. However, when relapse has been defined as the consumption of a single drink after treatment, relapse rates as high as 90% have been reported (Orford &

Edwards, 1977). Complicating this picture is the finding that drinking outcomes following treatment are highly variable. Many clients do not relapse, many who relapse do not do so immediately, and many who relapse do not remain relapsed (e.g., Annis & Ogborne, 1983; Moos et al., 1990; Polich, Armor, & Braiker, 1981).

While high rates of relapse following treatment are understandably discouraging, the data for months 3 through 12 are encouraging. Specifically, the rates of relapse between months 3 and 12 for clients who have not relapsed by month 3 are markedly lower than the rates during the first 3 months following treatment. This finding suggests the importance of preventing relapse immediately following treatment, given that the prospects for sustained abstinence are remarkably higher once an initial period of abstinence has been achieved.

In this chapter, we focus on the topics of relapse, relapse prevention, and dealing with relapses that do occur. We open with some important definitional issues, including attention to the distinction between a lapse and relapse. We then discuss relapse in the broader context of the stages of change model. We highlight the potential clinical advantages of conceptualizing relapse less as a discrete event and more as a process that can be influenced. The next section keys on issues surrounding the prevention and treatment of relapses. A case example will be used to describe strategies for addressing relapse issues in the treatment setting.

DEFINITIONS AND MODELS OF RELAPSE

Despite many years of consideration of the problem of relapse, relapse still is not operationally defined in any universally accepted way. However, there has been some progress in reaching consensus on a conceptual definition of relapse. In particular, there is agreement that it is important first to distinguish between a lapse and a relapse. A lapse is viewed as a single episode of violation of an individual's attempt at restraint. For example, a lapse might be a person's use of heroin during the first several months following his or her treatment for heroin addiction. Relapse, however, is more abstract than the neatly defined single event of a lapse and is seen in part as a psychological construct. Relapse is the reoccurrence of some problem after a period of improvement. Importantly, there is perception of a loss of control and a marking of the failure of a behavior change effort (Brownell, Marlatt, Lichtenstein, & Wilson, 1986; Shiffman, 1989).

A lapse does not necessarily lead to a relapse. It is essential to note, however, that, despite conceptual agreement to differentiate between lapse and relapse, the empirical literature frequently does not. Therefore, in describing or citing research we use the term "relapse" to cover both events, except where the authors distinguished between lapse and relapse.

There also has been considerable effort taken in recent years to develop models of relapse so as to help inform clinical practice and to guide future research. In this regard, Table 9.1 provides an overview of some of the more widely discussed models of relapse. The table covers only what we consider essential points about these models and is not meant to be a detailed review of them.

As Table 9.1 shows, the models and theories make few distinctions among different drugs as far as mechanisms of relapse are concerned. Also, the theories emphasize immediate relapse precipitants. Only the concept of "high-risk situation" could extend to more remote (from the relapse) events, but the idea of high risk is not clearly articulated. Furthermore, the theories could be divided into two general categories: psychological, with an emphasis on cognition (the first three theories in Table 9.1), and psychobiological (the last four theories in the table), with emphases on acquired motivation to use drugs and on urges and cravings. Within each of these classifications there is considerable overlap among theories. Except for the cognitive-behavioral and self-efficacy/outcome expectations approaches, the theories fail to differentiate between a lapse and a relapse.

Across the theories, there is a consistency in what they suggest should be assessed as being relevant to relapse events. The broadest content category is stimulus conditions that are thought to be antecedents of relapse. These may be internal or external events, depending on the theory. Therefore, mood (especially negative), physical state, and urges and cravings are identified as important relapse antecedents. "High-risk situations" may encompass any of these antecedents as well as other psychological, social, or physical elements that may lead to substance use. Note that the mechanisms hypothesized for how different stimulus conditions come to be antecedents of relapse differ among the theories, but the implications for measurement are similar.

The psychological theories require measurement of two types of expectancies. The first is outcome expectancies, which refer to the individual's beliefs about the effects of a drug if it is used in a given situation. The other type of expectancy is self-efficacy, or the individual's estimation that he or

TABLE 9.1. Summary of Major Models and Theories of Relapse

Model/theory	Mechanism(s) of relapse
Cognitive-behavioral model (Marlatt & Gordon, 1985)	Interaction between "high risk" (for substance use) and the individual's self-efficacy to cope with those situations without substance use determines relapse. Expectations about the utility of drugs and alcohol in a situation also are important. Cognitive and emotional processes represented by the "Abstinence Violation Effect" construct influence the severity and duration of relapse.
Person–situation interaction model (Litman, 1986)	Relapse is determined by an interaction among three factors: situations that the individual perceives as threatening ("high risk"), availability of an adequate repertoire of coping strategies, and the individual's perception of the appropriateness and effectiveness of available coping strategies.
Self-efficacy and outcome expectancies (Annis, 1986; Rollnick & Heather, 1982)	Initial substance use occurs from the mislabeling of negative affect and negative physical states as craving. After first substance use, expectations of control over such use decreases, along with self-efficacy. This process leads to a more severe relapse.
Opponent process (Solomon, 1980)	Through conditioning, formerly neutral internal and external stimuli become connected with various "A" and "B" states. Reexposure or reexperiencing these states may increase the individual's motivation to use drugs following a period of abstinence.
Craving and loss of control (Ludwig & Wikler, 1974)	Internal and external stimuli associated with drug withdrawal are labeled as craving. Drugs are sought as a way to relieve craving. Use of drugs then leads to a loss of control, due to inaccurate interpretation of interoceptive cues that regulate consumption.
Urges and craving (Tiffany, 1990, 1992; Wise, 1988)	Drug use and drug urges and cravings have occurred enough times to be "automatic cognitive processes." In the abstinent substance abuser, these processes can be triggered by various internal and external stimuli. Relapse may occur if an adequate "action plan" not to use drugs, a nonautomatic cognitive process, is impeded or not used. Wise adds that use of one drug may trigger urges to use another, a result of action in the brain.

TABLE 9.1. (continued)

Model/theory	Mechanism(s) of relapse
Post-acute withdrawal syndrome (Gorski & Miller, 1979)	Relapse is defined as a "process that occurs within the patient which manifests itself in a progressive pattern of behavior that allows the symptoms of a disease or illness to become reactivated in a person that has previously arrested those symptoms" (Gorski & Miller, 1979, p. 1). The model, developed in the context of alcohol use disorders, focuses primarily on the physiological and neurological effects of the substance on the user. When the user seeks to abstain, he or she initially goes through a period of withdrawal. This is followed by what Gorski and Miller term "Post Acute Withdrawal Syndrome (PAW)," which primarily affects higher-level cognitive functioning (e.g., abstract thinking, memory) and is linked to higher levels of emotionality and overreaction to stress. The relapse process itself follows a consistent pattern. First, the individual's attitude changes as he or she begins to question his or her well-being and ability to stay sober. The individual begins to use maladaptive coping methods, resulting in negative emotional consequences. The end result of this process is a resumption of use.

Note. Adapted from Donovan and Chaney (1985); Connors, Maisto, and Donovan (1996); and original sources.

she can successfully enact a behavior in a given situation. Finally, psychological theories require the assessment of the individual's pattern of coping in different situations that may be related to substance use.

The most discussed model of the relapse process has been provided by Marlatt and his colleagues (summarized in Marlatt & Gordon, 1985). The basic model is shown in Figure 9.2. Marlatt hypothesized that the initiation of abstinence engenders a sense of personal control and self-efficacy, self-perceptions that become strengthened as the period of abstinence lengthens. Over this period, the substance abuser is likely to face situations that put him or her at risk for again using alcohol or drugs. Such "high-risk" situations are a central feature of the Marlatt model of relapse. The antecedents to such situations can be varied, but frequently they reflect cognitive and lifestyle factors that subsequently can place the person in a high-risk situation. When a person is placed in such a situation, the ideal response would be an effective coping behavior. When such a behavior is in the person's behavioral repertoire and is emitted,

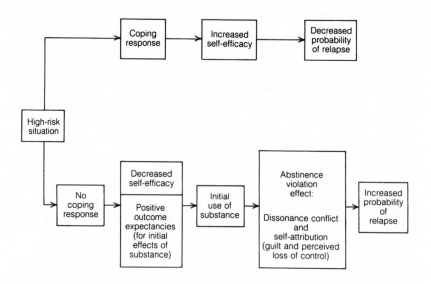

FIGURE 9.2. The Marlatt and Gordon model of the relapse process. From Marlatt (1985b, p. 38). Copyright 1985 by The Guilford Press. Reprinted by permission.

then the success experience enhances the person's self-efficacy (Bandura, 1977). This, in turn, decreases the probability of relapse in similar subsequent situations. On the other hand, if the person is unable to emit an effective coping response, then this will lead to a decreased level of self-efficacy and an increase in the attractiveness of the substance as a mechanism for dealing with the situation. This is particularly the case if the person maintains positive outcome expectancies regarding drug effects. As the attractiveness of the substance increases (in conjunction with decreased self-efficacy), it becomes more likely that the person will use the drug in that situation. If the drug is used, an abstinence violation effect (AVE) will result, involving dissonance frequently accompanied by self-attributions of guilt and low self-esteem, both of which can propel an initial use of the substance into a full-blown relapse.

One of the hallmark features of the Marlatt model is the high-risk situation. According to Cummings, Gordon, and Marlatt (1980), "high-risk situations are associated with a history of use of the addictive behavior as a coping response and thus represent a critical choice point for the individual" (p. 297). As such, high-risk situations often serve as precipitants to relapse to substance use. In order to test this notion, Marlatt and Gordon (1980) performed a content analysis of situations associated with relapse. Using their schema, relapse situations were coded into two broad categories. The first represented intrapersonal–environmental determinants, which include determinants associated primarily with within-person factors and/or reactions to nonpersonal environmental events. The five subcategories of intrapersonal–environmental determinants were coping with negative emotional states, coping with negative physical-physiological states, enhancement of positive emotional states, testing personal control, or giving in to temptations or urges. The second broad category represented interpersonal determinants, which include factors associated with interpersonal events. The subcategories within this group were coping with interpersonal conflict, social pressure, and enhancement of positive emotional states. Table 9.2 provides a breakdown of the high-risk situations described by several groups of substance abusers. As shown, the majority of alcoholics attributed relapse to intrapersonal determinants (61% of the relapse situations). Predominant within this category were situations involving negative emotional states, such as frustration or anger.

TABLE 9.2. Analysis of Relapse Situations among Alcoholics, Smokers, and Heroin Addicts

Relapse situation	Frequency		
	Alcoholics	Smokers	Heroin addicts
Intrapersonal determinants			
Negative emotional states	38%	37%	19%
Negative physical states	3%	2%	9%
Positive emotional states	—	6%	10%
Testing personal control	9%	—	2%
Urges and temptations	11%	5%	5%
Total	61%	50%	45%
Interpersonal determinants			
Interpersonal conflict	18%	15%	14%
Social pressure	18%	32%	36%
Positive emotional states	3%	3%	5%
Total	39%	50%	55%

Note. Adapted from Marlatt (1985b, p. 39). Copyright 1985 by The Guilford Press. Adapted by permission.

The remaining relapse situations among alcoholics (39%) included inter-personal determinants, especially interpersonal conflicts and social pressure. The relapse situations for smokers and heroin addicts differed in several ways from those reported by the alcoholics. The smokers and heroin addicts reported a lower percentage of relapses with intrapersonal determinants. This was predominantly attributable to relatively fewer endorsements of testing personal control and urges and temptations and relatively greater endorsements of positive emotional states as relapse precipitants. The smokers and heroin addicts also reported a greater frequency of interpersonal determinants, relative to the alcoholics. This difference was almost entirely attributable to the smokers and heroin addicts reporting social pressure as a relapse precipitant at a rate double that of the alcoholics. Thirty-two percent of the relapses described by smokers and 36% of those described by the heroin addicts were attributed to social pressure. The only other differences of note were between the smokers and heroin addicts. The smokers described negative emotional states as a precipitant almost twice as often as the heroin addicts (37% vs. 19%), while the heroin addicts described negative physical states as a precipitant more often than the smokers (9% vs. 2%).

The pattern of findings noted above for relapse precipitants has been reported for other groups as well. Wallace (1989), for example, assessed psychological and environmental determinants of relapse among crack cocaine smokers. She found that the most frequent precursors to relapses were painful emotional states (40% of relapses), failure to enter aftercare following treatment (37%), and encounters with conditioned environment stimuli (34%). In another report, Birke, Edelmann, and Davis (1990) found among illicit drug users that the most important relapse precipitants were negative affect and interpersonal conflict (but not social pressure).

While the studies described above identify types of scenarios in which relapses are likely to occur, note that there are strong indications that relapses are not precipitated by particular factors but instead that multiple influences can operate simultaneously in leading to a relapse. This was clearly indicated by Wallace (1989). In that study, specific precipitants of relapses were identified, such as painful emotional states. However, Wallace also found that the great majority of relapses (86%) actually were multidetermined. That is, in most cases two or more categories of precipitants were acting together to set the stage for the relapse, at least among crack cocaine smokers. A similar finding has been reported by Heather, Stallard, and Tebbutt (1991) and Zywiak, Connors, Maisto, and Westerberg (1996); in each case, it was found that combinations of relapse precipitants typically operate in the context of a particular relapse event.

RELAPSE IN THE BROADER CONTEXT
OF THE STAGES OF CHANGE MODEL

We noted earlier, in Chapter 1, that a basic feature of the stages of change model is that it is cyclic. A person more often will go back to an earlier stage of change after reaching a later one, generally as a result of a lapse or relapse. Such reversions (for example, a person in action relapsing and reverting to contemplation) are generally viewed as setbacks, although the person seeking to change in most cases does not revert back to the precontemplation stage. Although individuals often relapse during the action stage, the problem of relapse is most often conceptualized and discussed in the context of the maintenance stage.

While relapse is not a stage in the stages of change model, it nevertheless is an important and relevant clinical issue. As noted above, clients often move back in the stage sequence as a result of a relapse. Indeed, it is not uncommon for several such reversions to occur before a durable behavioral change pattern has been established (Prochaska & DiClemente, 1986). In this context, relapses might well be viewed as an expected event in the overall change process. While a relapse can lead to a reversion back to the precontemplation stage, it is encouraging to note that the vast majority of regressions are to the contemplation or preparation stages (Prochaska & DiClemente, 1984).

A final point on why relapses are relevant to the stages of change model is that they can be viewed as the flip side of the maintenance stage. As such, a major task for the person in the maintenance stage is to avoid relapsing.

MAINTAINING ABSTINENCE
AND ADDRESSING RELAPSE

For clients who have moved through the action stage and into maintenance, the overarching objective is the consolidation and maintenance of gains. This, of course, entails the avoidance of relapse and the mini-mization of relapses, should they occur. Accordingly, this section on treat-ment issues focuses on two topics. The first is maintaining treatment gains (typically maintaining abstinence) and thus preventing relapse. The sec-ond topic is addressing relapses that do occur.

Maintaining Treatment Gains and Preventing Relapses

While relapse is perhaps the most common outcome following substance abuse treatment, there are individuals who achieve abstinence and main-tain it for extended periods. In a recent national study evaluating the re-sponse of alcoholics to different treatments, for example, 19% of the cli-ents seen as outpatients and 35% of the clients treated in aftercare (following a more intensive inpatient or day hospital program) were ab-stinent throughout a 1-year follow-up period (Project MATCH Re-search Group, 1997a).

How is it that clients maintain durable periods of abstinence? One line of clinical research addressing this question concerns client-identified factors associated with their periods of abstinence. Two recent studies have provided some insights on these factors. In the first, McKay, Maisto, and O'Farrell (1996) interviewed male alcoholics periodically over a 30-month period following alcohol treatment that included behavioral mar-ital therapy. At each follow-up contact, the client was asked about factors associated with any 30-day (or longer) period of continuous abstinence during the follow-up interval being assessed. Factors reflecting what were conceptualized as "active strategies" consistently emerged across each follow-up interview. In this regard, the predominant strategies were re-calling the benefits of sobriety, recalling drinking problems, and remem-bering that sobriety is the first priority. In a second study, men and women alcoholics were similarly interviewed about factors associated with posttreatment abstinence (Connors, Maisto, & Zywiak, 1998). The methods for maintaining abstinence used most frequently (used in over 60% of the abstinent periods by both men and women) were avoiding risky people and places, recalling drinking-related problems, treatment, and self-help groups. Also used frequently by both men and women were the strategies of staying in alcohol-free environments, using treatment skills, avoiding thinking about alcohol, recalling the benefits of sobriety, and remembering sobriety as the top priority. The only difference be-tween men and women on the endorsement of these factors as an aid in maintaining abstinence was on the method of recalling drinking problems. That strategy was used in 80% of the abstinent periods among men and in 61% of the periods among the women.

These two studies taken together suggest that clients, after treatment, use a variety of strategies in the service of maintaining abstinence. Importantly, men and women for the most part used these strategies to a comparable extent. Some specific clinical issues related to relapse, and associated clinical responses, were described earlier in Chapter 5.

Further information on the issue of maintaining abstinence has emerged from research on predictors of abstinence and other dimensions of positive posttreatment functioning. Not surprisingly, there are a considerable number of strong indications that cognitive coping skills, positive thinking, and number of available coping skills are all related to posttreatment abstinence (Litman, Eiser, Rawson, & Oppenheim, 1979; McKay, Maisto, et al., 1996; Moos, Finney, & Cronkite, 1990). In a recent prospective investigation of posttreatment functioning, with a particular focus on relapse events, Miller, Westerberg, Harris, and Tonigan (1996) found that clients' coping skills were a powerful predictor of treatment outcome. More specifically, positive coping skills were associated with less subsequent drinking and avoidant coping styles predicted relapse. Similarly, Connors, Maisto, and Zywiak (1996) found that coping skills and responses generally (including available coping behaviors and perceived self-efficacy regarding the use of such behaviors) predicted a host of posttreatment outcomes (including a greater percentage of days abstinent, fewer drinking consequences, and fewer craving experiences).

These two lines of clinical research—survey assessments of factors associated with periods of abstinence and the identification of variables that are predictive of posttreatment functioning—converge in highlighting the role of active coping behaviors in maintaining abstinence and avoiding relapsing. Relatedly, treatments with the strongest evidence of efficacy prominently include those focused on developing and/or applying coping skills and altering social relationships (Miller et al., 1995).

The foregoing research also provides some guidance for helping clients set the stage for maintaining abstinence. For starters, clients should be aware of the techniques and strategies used by others to maintain abstinence, such as recalling problems associated with past drinking, participating in self-help groups, and avoiding risky people and places. Clients should identify factors associated with any of their own periods of previous abstinence, should there be such a history. The counselor and client can then focus on those strategies that appear most applicable to the client's unique needs and circumstances. It is often useful for clients to have these strategies listed on a card for their frequent review.

A key part of avoiding relapse is identifying situations in which the client is at greater risk for relapse. We presented an array of such situations earlier in this chapter. In the clinical setting, it will help to have clients identify scenarios in which they are vulnerable to substance use, either based on previous substance use patterns or anticipated situations in the immediate future. Such assessments should be conducted using open-ended questioning about high-risk situations and/or using measures specifically developed to assess domains of situations in which the client is more likely to use alcohol or drugs, such as the Situational Confidence Questionnaire (Annis, 1982b) for alcohol and the Drug-Taking Confidence Questionnaire (Annis & Martin, 1985) for other drug use (described in Chapter 3). Among outpatient alcohol abusers, for example, higher confidence to avoid drinking, assessed using the Alcohol Abstinence Self-Efficacy Scale (AASE), is associated with better treatment outcomes (Project MATCH Research Group, 1997b). Relatedly, the relationship between temptation to drink and confidence to not drink was another predictor of outcome. Clients with greater confidence relative to temptation on the AASE reported more posttreatment abstinent days and fewer drinks per drinking day. Thus, evaluating and addressing both temptations and confidence appear to be important in maximizing prospects of avoiding relapses.

Finally, a third clinical implication is to focus on the development and application of coping skills generally and especially those with relevance to high-risk situations. Interestingly, research by Miller et al. (1996) suggests that client coping skills determined the avoidance of relapse—independent of the overall amount of stress and risk to which the client was exposed. As such, treatment providers may want to incorporate into their standard practices coping skills assessment and training, should that not already be part of the treatments being offered. Among the available resources on coping skills training for substance abusers are those by Monti et al. (1989) and Kadden et al. (1992).

The foregoing interventions are intended to maximize client awareness of and sensitivity to behaviors associated with abstinence and scenarios that represent heightened risk for substance use. This endeavor has the potential for placing the client in the best position possible for productively using coping and other life functioning skills to maintain abstinence in particular but more generally to support and engender a positive and gratifying lifestyle (see Marlatt, 1985a, for a more general discussion on lifestyle modification).

Addressing Relapses

Most clients will experience a relapse in some form. While not desirable events, relapses nevertheless can be constructively used clinically in the service of reachieving abstinence for a longer period. In this regard, relapses should be framed as learning experiences, if and when they occur. Accordingly, in this section on addressing relapses we focus on preparing clients to deal with and terminate relapse episodes and reengaging the client in the change process.

Preparing Clients to Deal with and Terminate Relapses

The various high-risk scenarios in which relapse might occur for a given client were described earlier in this chapter. Ideally, client sensitivity to such situations and awareness and use of strategies to cope with these situations will preclude relapse for many. However, for those who do relapse, the ideal response on the part of the client will be to take steps immediately to minimize the extent of substance use and interrupt the relapse process.

Contingency plans for dealing with a relapse should be developed as part of treatment and before an actual relapse. Examples of behaviors a client might seek to engage in would include leaving the substance use environment, contacting one's counselor or sponsor, reinitiating self-help group attendance, and so on. Often counselors have their clients develop a written list of things to do if a relapse occurs and have them keep it in their wallets for ready access. An example of such a list is shown in Table 9.3.

Reengaging the Client in the Change Process

Assuming the client's response to the relapse leads to a return to treatment, the counselor's tasks are similar to those faced when initiating treatment more generally. A first step would be an assessment of the client's current status in terms of substance use and immediate risk for subsequent use. Client stabilization and resolution of the relapse (if still in progress) is the most pressing clinical need. Dovetailing with this would be an assessment of the client's current stage of change. If the client was

TABLE 9.3. Reference Sheet for Use by Clients

What to do if a relapse occurs

1. Use the relapse as a learning experience.

2. See the relapse as a specific, unique event.

3. Examine the relapse openly in order to reduce the amount of guilt and/or shame you may feel (those thoughts can lead to a feeling of hopelessness and continued drinking).

4. Analyze the triggers for the relapse.

5. Examine what the expectations about drinking were at the time (what did you anticipate drinking would accomplish in that situation?).

6. Plan for dealing with the aftermath/consequences of the relapse.

7. Tell yourself that control is only a moment away.

8. Renew your commitment to abstinence.

9. Make immediate plans for recovery—don't hesitate, do it now!

10. Contact your counselor and discuss slips.

in the maintenance stage, has he or she cycled back to contemplation—thinking about change but not acting yet? If so, interventions intended to move the client from contemplation to action would be warranted.

Regardless of the stage to which the client has cycled back, therapists should continue to use the motivational counseling techniques described earlier (in Chapter 2). In addition, attention should be placed on the reestablishment of those techniques and strategies previously used by the client to achieve and maintain abstinent periods in the past. Naturally, it may be instructive to review these techniques and strategies in light of the circumstances surrounding the relapse. Finally, supplemental treatment interventions may be necessary to address problem areas that have been exacerbated or have newly arisen as a function of the recent substance use.

CASE EXAMPLE OF A CLIENT WHO HAS RELAPSED

Angela M is now a 48-year-old woman who had achieved 21 months of sobriety, following a period of problematic drinking that extended over two decades.

Angela's background and drinking history were described earlier, in

Chapter 2, in the context of a case example of a person in the maintenance stage. Briefly, Angela described a long-term problem with drinking that was characterized by a variety of negative consequences, including a pair of arrests for driving under the influence of alcohol. She also participated in treatment programs on several occasions, with some limited improvements experienced.

Angela's third course of outpatient treatment "took hold"—largely, she felt, because she was resolved to abstain completely and because she had a strong working relationship with her counselor. Her treatment sessions focused on a variety of strategies for achieving durable abstinence, developing alternatives to drinking (including stress management, avoiding situations associated with previous heavy drinking, coping with cravings and urges, and drink refusal skills), including Peter, her husband of 10 years, in portions of treatment to incorporate his support and encouragement, and developing plans to prevent relapse or at least to minimize drinking should a slip occur.

While she experienced some setbacks during the first 10 months of treatment, Angela generally rebounded quickly and, perhaps more importantly, felt she had learned valuable "sobriety lessons" from such events. Angela had incorporated a variety of change strategies that she had been using successfully, following an early period of trial and error in the application of these strategies. Now her attention was focused on what she called "cruise control," whereby she could step back from the vigilance associated with skills acquisition and application and instead let much of that behavior occur more naturally. She emphasized that "cruise control" still entailed paying close attention to her environment, including attention to her own thoughts and feelings. Further, Angela still spent time anticipating drinking situations and reviewed beforehand her plans to deal with such situations. She still experienced periodic thoughts and temptations regarding alcohol use, although she was pleased that she could not really classify them as cravings. Finally, it was Angela's sense that she would always need to be in a state of full awareness regarding potential challenges to her abstinence and that she would never be in a position to take her sobriety for granted.

Angela's contacts with her therapist tapered off, and she terminated treatment shortly after achieving 14 months of continuous abstinence. Seven months later she recontacted her counselor to return to treatment. Angela had relapsed and had been drinking heavily again over the preceding 2 months.

At her next session with her counselor, Angela reported that she had been doing fine during the first several months after her last treatment session. She had been doing well on her job, and her relationship with Peter continued to be positive and rewarding. The only domain in which she felt something was lacking concerned friendships. She noted that she had no close friends and relatively few acquaintances, either at work or outside work. Angela felt she had good working relationships with her coworkers but that the relationships did not extend beyond that context.

Around 4 months before returning to treatment, Angela was approached by a job "headhunter" about taking a position at a large, established company on the other side of town. She was flattered by the inquiry and decided to interview for the position. Angela afterward evaluated the advantages and disadvantages or unknowns about the new position. On the positive side, the job offered new challenges and opportunities for professional growth and advancement. It also included a significant increase in salary. The main disadvantage was leaving a relatively comfortable position where she was productive and content. Angela ultimately decided to accept the position for two reasons: the opportunities for advancement and for new social contacts. This latter advantage came to the forefront of her deliberations because she was continuing to feel the need to develop some close friendships, which were not emerging at her current job.

The job transition was a difficult one. Angela experienced almost immediately an increased level of pressure to perform, a greater workload, longer work hours, and a much more competitive environment. These combined forces resulted in a heightened general level of stress and a significant decrease in the amount of time and energy she had available for her relationship with Peter (although she reported him to be supportive of her during this difficult time). Despite these intimidations, Angela reported that she felt her work performance was satisfactory. Indeed, she found it "heady" to be working in an upscale company she felt was on the "cutting edge" of her profession. In addition, she found herself more socially involved with her coworkers than she had been at her previous place of employment. Unfortunately, although she did not immediately recognize it, most of these contacts occurred in settings where alcohol was available and used widely. For example, it was not uncommon for her coworkers to have a beer or glass of wine with lunch or dinner, and heavier drinking typically occurred at bars after work.

Angela reported that not drinking at lunch was easy. She did, however, feel more pressure internally as well as externally to drinking with her coworkers after work. The external pressures revolved around situations where someone would offer her a drink or buy a round of drinks for the group. She was, among these individuals, the only non-drinker (at that point). The internal pressures were more complicated. On the one hand, she felt she shouldn't be drinking or even thinking about it. On the other hand, she felt she was in pretty solid control of her life and that drinking in a circumscribed setting would not only be manageable but also help her fit in more with her colleagues and perhaps also better set the stage for developing the friendships she was seeking. It was on this basis that she indeed did start drinking again. Initially she drank only at the "happy hour" sessions, finding—somewhat to her surprise, she reports now—that she was able to keep it "under control." She felt she was drinking more than she should, but that it was not "really out of hand" in the eyes of the others. However, she unexpectedly found herself drinking much more when alone at home, especially when Peter was out, and it was this drinking that was causing the most tangible consequences for her. In this regard, she was becoming inconsistent in getting to work on time, she felt "fuzzy" during the first couple of hours, and she perceived a withdrawal on the part of Peter from their relationship. It was this cluster of concerns, especially the concern about the relationship with Peter, that led to Angela's decision to recontact her therapist. In addition, she was realizing gradually that her drinking in the social contexts was not leading to the development of friendships with her coworkers.

An assessment of Angela's recent drinking indicated that she was drinking with her coworkers after work around 3 days per week, typically Tuesday, Thursday, and Friday. On these occasions, she was typically consuming around three to five glasses of wine over a 2- or 3-hour period, depending on the day. At home Angela was generally consuming around three to four glasses of wine most weekday evenings, a glass or so less on evenings she was out earlier with her coworkers. She also drank on weekend days, although more sporadically; when Peter was not around, she was drinking more over the course of the day. Angela's drinking predominantly had the effect of dulling most of her senses, which was not an entirely unwelcome consequence to her.

At her return session, Angela verbalized a desire to reestablish abstinence. Over the several days before her session she had ceased drinking. Her evaluation of the pros and cons of drinking led her to this decision. The pros she had anticipated when she decided to return to drinking had not materialized—she did not fit in better with her coworkers and closer friendships did not emerge. The cons of drinking that were most striking to her at this point were the hungover feelings at work and the distancing exhibited by her husband. Further, she had not anticipated the home-bound drinking that emerged, added drinking that she felt was physically depressing her. Angela reported that she was ready to quit, and that indeed she had initiated action on this endeavor several days before. She felt the challenge before her in terms of drinking was to not relapse.

Angela's counselor devoted much of their session to a review of events since their last sessions, focusing on the time since the return to drinking. The counselor utilized a variety of the strategies described earlier in this volume in the context of motivational counseling. In the present case, Angela had determined that she wanted to continue the abstinence initiated several days earlier. They focused on the strategies utilized by Angela earlier to achieve abstinence and maintain it for over a year. For Angela, one of the strongest motivations for remaining abstinent was the recognition and continuing awareness that the resumption of drinking yielded none of the expected positives and resulted in several unanticipated negative consequences. The session keyed on here-and-now strategies, all action-oriented, for continuing the abstinence begun and for avoiding drinking and drinking-related situations during the upcoming week. In this regard, Angela determined to continue her luncheons with coworkers, where she had not been drinking, and terminate, at least for the time being, the "happy hour" excursions. This would allow continuing contact with coworkers but would be confined to a safer context. She also sought to exert more structure to her evenings, where she had gotten into the habit of drinking. Part of this structuring effort was to include planned activities, either in the house or outside, with Peter during those occasions when he was available. Finally, it was agreed at this session that subsequent sessions would focus first and foremost on maintaining abstinence and avoiding relapse, and also on developing a plan for evaluating and addressing as warranted other issues related to Angela's overall life-functioning, including the development of closer friendships.

SUMMARY

- Relapse refers to a return to substance use following a period of abstinence. Relapses are a common posttreatment phenomenon.
- A variety of models and theories have been developed to account for the relapse process. Most emphasize immediate relapse precipitants.
- Several studies have identified a number of interpersonal and intrapersonal factors as primary determinants of relapses. However, relapses are perhaps more productively evaluated as being the result of multiple influences operating simultaneously.
- While a relapse can lead to a reversion back to the precontemplation stage of change, most regressions are to the contemplation or preparation stages.
- Studies assessing strategies used by abstinent substance abusers to maintain abstinence may provide guidance to clients seeking durable abstinence. These strategies include recalling the benefits of sobriety, recalling drinking problems, and avoiding risky people and places.
- There are strong indications that cognitive coping skills, positive thinking, and having a number of available coping skills are all related to posttreatment abstinence.
- When clients return to treatment following a relapse, the classical priorities are terminating the relapse episode and reengaging the client in the change process.
- While not desirable events, relapses nevertheless should be constructively used clinically in the service of reachieving abstinence for a longer period of time.

10

FINAL THOUGHTS
AND FUTURE DIRECTIONS

The idea that behavior change is complex and involves a path or process is not new. Therapists and counselors from many different theoretical orientations have described complex mechanisms to promote change (see Prochaska & Norcross, 1999). These include making the unconscious conscious (Freud), removing conditions of worth (Rogers), employing various schedules of reinforcement (Skinner), emotional release (Perls), and shifting family systems (Minuchin). All theories describe defenses and barriers that make change problematic. Most identify critical moments or incidents that foster change and involve insight, behavior, or emotions. Some theories target global problems (the Oedipus complex, meaning, self-actualization) and others concentrate on behavior-specific problems (fear of flying, panic attacks). However, all acknowledge the difficulty of achieving long-term successful change. These different theories give direction to our current substance abuse treatments and demonstrate the complexity of the problems and the process involved in changing behavior.

Over the past 30 years, a series of clinical trial research studies have compared treatments from very different theories to see which one was superior to the others. This "horse race" research design has not found a single specific treatment for substance abuse that consistently does better than all the others. Most psychosocial treatments beat the control entries in the race but finish in a dead heat against one another (Luborsky, Singer, & Luborsky, 1975). Recent trials in substance abuse treatment have demonstrated similar results. The Collaborative Cocaine Treatment Study showed little difference among the different treatment conditions (Crits-Christoph et al., 1999). Project MATCH, a large treatment matching trial, demonstrated similar outcomes among three treatments that differed significantly in intensity and in philosophy (Project MATCH Research Group, 1997a, 1997b, 1998a). There is a growing consensus that common elements or a common path of change may underlie all treatments (Norcross & Goldfried, 1992). Even the NIMH depression trial that compared medication with two types of psychotherapy (interpersonal and cognitive) found that there were few differences in long-term outcomes with these very different types of treatments (Elkin et al., 1989). This body of research points to the importance of some common elements that operate across all treatments. Some researchers have identified commonalities in the treatment relationship, therapist variables, or client variables as the source of the common outcomes (Beutler & Clarkin, 1990). However, it seems equally plausible that the common element across treatments is how they interact with the process of change that we have highlighted in this book.

The stages of change model can be both integrative and eclectic. The model offers neither a theory of personality nor an extensive exposition of the biopsychosocial factors that contribute to the development of the problem. The focus of the model is the identification of important components that are common to the change process, whether that change occurs with or without the aid of formal treatment (Prochaska & DiClemente, 1983, 1984; DiClemente & Prochaska, 1998). The model grew out of early attempts to look across systems of psychotherapy to find common processes of change (Prochaska, 1979) and became more explicit in the exploration of addictive behaviors and other types of psychopathology (DiClemente & Prochaska, 1982, 1985; Prochaska & DiClemente, 1982, 1984; Prochaska et al., 1992).

Development of this model was influenced by many of the discoveries and dilemmas uncovered by researchers in both psychotherapy and addiction from 1950 to 1980. During the 1970s, there was growing interest in how attitudes and decision making influenced behavior change

(Janis & Mann, 1977). Behavior therapy and behavior modification increased awareness that identifying and concentrating on specific behaviors could increase the effectiveness of our treatments (Craighead, Craighead, & Ilardi, 1995). These trends led to the growth of the social learning perspective and the development of cognitive-behavior therapy (Bandura, 1986; Meichenbaum, 1995). In addition, there was growing recognition of the problem of relapse in addictive behaviors (Brownell et al., 1986). Once treatment researchers began including long-term follow-up of treated clients, practitioners realized that maintenance of behavior change did not automatically follow short-term success (Marlatt & Gordon, 1985; Brownell et al., 1986). In the area of smoking cessation and alcoholism treatment, in particular, there was growing awareness that knowledge, education, and social support were necessary but not sufficient to produce behavior change (Glynn, Boyd, & Gruman, 1990). Relapse was a persistent and rather intractable problem (Lichtenstein, 1971). As the complexity and multiple aspects of change became clearer, some researchers began to delineate distinguishable steps or tasks that were involved in creating sustained change of addictive behaviors (Horn, 1976; DiClemente & Prochaska, 1982).

The increasing eclecticism among therapists and the growing insight into the process of change laid the foundation for the development of the stages of change model. The model offered an understandable and clinically useful perspective on the process of change. These stages divided up the process of change into segments that highlighted the critical issues of denial, decision making, anticipation, action, relapse, and maintenance for specific behavioral problems. This wide-angle view of the process of change was the initial insight that caught the attention of therapists and counselors and gave them a terminology to describe their experiences with clients in treatment. Treatment professionals from New England to New Zealand and from Scotland to South Africa began to use the terminology and to recognize clients as being in precontemplation or contemplation for change, rather than expecting all of them to be either ready for action or in denial. That this process of change was cyclical and not linear was another concept that appeared to be completely in synch with the experiences of addiction counselors and therapists. Stages of change and recycling through these stages highlighted not only where the client was at a particular point in time but where the client had been in terms of his or her change history. The ability of the stages to capture descriptively what many therapists experienced accounts for the initial success and spread of the stages of change construct (Joseph, Breslin, & Skinner, 1999).

In addition to being a useful descriptive, the stages have also proved to be useful in predicting the attendance, participation, and progress of clients in changing problem behaviors or in beginning health protection behaviors (DiClemente & Prochaska, 1998). There is growing evidence that stage status or readiness to change is a solid predictor of treatment participation (Smith et al., 1995), of behavior change in the natural environment without formal treatment (DiClemente & Prochaska, 1985), and of treatment outcomes (Project MATCH Research Group, 1997a, 1998a). However, not every study comes up with identical results, and more research and thinking need to be devoted to explaining the differences in research findings.

What has been most interesting in the research findings about stages of change is that stage status is reliably related to the types of change mechanisms or coping activities that have been labeled processes of change. Evidence from a number of studies indicates that cognitive and experiential processes of change are differentially important in the early stages and behavioral processes more important in the later stages of change (Prochaska et al., 1991; Perz et al., 1996; Chapter 1 of this volume). Behavioral processes of change increase in frequency as individuals move through the preparation, action, and maintenance stages. Certain processes, like self-reevaluation, increase in the earlier stages of change and then decrease during action and maintenance (DiClemente & Prochaska, 1985). The interaction of the stages and processes of change across multiple problem behaviors offers critical support for the integrative and comprehensive nature of this model. If stage of change were not related to coping activities and other markers of change like decisional balance and self-efficacy, stages would simply represent descriptive labels offering little or no direction for treatment.

CLINICAL UTILITY OF THE STAGES OF CHANGE MODEL

A significant contribution of the model is the identification of different tasks and challenges that face the client and the therapist at different points in the process of changing addictive behaviors (Miller & Rollnick, 1991; DiClemente, 1991; DiClemente & Prochaska, 1998). We highlight below several key contributions of the stages of change model to the treatment of substance abuse. Clinical utility of this model derives from the clarification of the role of the client in the process of change, recognition of critical stage-specific tasks for client and therapist, and identification of the cyclical and spiral nature of the process of change.

Role of the Client

If there is a common process of intentional human behavior change, it should be essentially the same when individuals change a problem behavior with or without formal treatment (DiClemente & Prochaska, 1982, 1998). Studies that have examined self-change as well as those that have concentrated on treatment seekers have uncovered many similarities in terms of this process of change (Sobell, Cunningham, Sobell, & Toneatto, 1993; Klingemann, 1991; Tucker et al., 1995; DiClemente & Prochaska, 1985; DiClemente, Carbonari, Zweben, et al., 2001). In reality the client is in charge of the change process since it begins well before he or she enters treatment and does not end with the completion of treatment (DiClemente & Prochaska, 1998; DiClemente, 1999a).

The therapist role has been described as a coach or midwife to this unfolding process of change (DiClemente, 1991). The client is seen as having responsibility for moving from one stage to another and for using the process of change that would foster movement through the stages of change to attain successful recovery. However, responsibility is not the same as blame. Having an important role in the process of change is not equivalent to the moral model view of substance abuse that blames clients for the problem and orders them to clean up their act and change (Donovan & Marlatt, 1988).

The perspective of the stages of change highlights that there are multiple tasks encountered on the road to recovery from addiction and that the process of change is a difficult one requiring effort and energy on the part of the client. Many individuals have difficulty making the change that leads to recovery. From the stages perspective some clients appear not to know what to do. Others seem to have insufficient motivation and other life problems. Still others appear to be trying too hard with inadequate assistance or ineffective strategies. Although the process is a complicated one, it is the client who must ultimately become motivated, make decisions, create a plan, and follow through on that plan in order for the substance abuse behavior to change.

Critical Tasks for Client and Therapist

Although the client is in charge of the change process, the therapist is not simply an idle bystander or an authoritarian figure who can order the client into action. A therapist cannot make a client change, but he or she can support or interfere with the process of change (Project MATCH Research Group, 1998b; DiClemente, 1999a). Treatments and therapists are not inert, inactive elements in the process of change. Their responsibility seems to be to instigate and support the process of change. However, they are not responsible for implementing the required tasks and activities needed to move through the process (Tucker et al., 1995). Treatments and therapists are catalysts that can create the atmosphere for change and can contribute important elements to the behavior change process. But the therapist does not *make* the change happen. The stages of change model provides a perspective on the process of change that offers a roadmap to the therapist. The roadmap indicates what to do to assist the client to move forward through the stages, through the cycle of change, to achieve successful, sustained recovery from the substance abuse problem.

As we have described in detail in previous chapters, there are specific tasks and challenges related to moving forward for each of the stages of change. The ideal treatment matching would be to have the therapist and the client consciously collaborating on the same goals and tasks that are required at each stage in the process. If the counselor or therapist is offering action options when the client is in precontemplation, treatment will fail. Since it is the client who needs to change the drug and alcohol dependence, it is the client's process of change that must be accurately tracked. Hence, knowing the location of the client in the process of change and using that knowledge to guide the selection of intervention goals and strategies are both critical.

The Cyclical and Spiral Nature of Change

The stages of change model's characterization of the flow of the process of change as a spiral also has proved helpful to clinicians. Addictions are complicated habits involving biological, psychological, and environmental components. As clients become addicted, they learn how to access, use, and hide their drugs of choice. They modify their lives to accommodate the substance abuse. Thus, there is an important learning component to the creation of these habits. There is also a learning component to the modification of these habits (DiClemente, 1999a; Donovan & Marlatt, 1988; Rotgers, Keller, & Morgenstern, 1996; Tucker et al., 1995; Werch & DiClemente, 1994). Substance abusers must learn how problematic their drug or alcohol problems are, what the pros and cons are for change, how firm a commitment to make, what strategies to use, and how to change their lives to eliminate those behaviors. These things are not ordinarily learned in a single day or in a single successful attempt to change. False starts and relapse are part of the learning process. Recycling through the stages appears to be a normal part of the process of recovery. However, the cycling should not be endless. Rapid and unproductive cycling through the stages indicates a serious problem in the process of change (Carbonari, DiClemente, & Sewell, 1999; DiClemente & Prochaska, 1998; DiClemente & Scott, 1997). Recycling, at its most productive, is a learning process wherein the individual and the therapist learn what will and will not work for that individual to change successfully. Thus, the process is described as a spiral one in which the client moves through the stages repeatedly until he or she reaches sustained change. This notion apparently has brought comfort and direction to many clients and therapists, enabling them to reconceptualize the work of breaking away from addictions in a more realistic and helpful manner.

Despite its contributions to clinical practice in treating addictive behaviors, the stages of change model raises many interesting questions that are only beginning to be researched since it has face validity but begs for additional confirmation or disconfirmation of its components.

EVALUATING CURRENT STATUS AND CRITIQUES OF THE STAGES OF CHANGE MODEL

The widespread use of the stages and processes of change in the treatment of addictive behaviors has not been uniformly well received. Some clinicians and researchers have expressed concerns about the model and its utility (Bandura, 1997; Davidson, 1992; Farkas et al., 1996; Pierce, Farkas, Zhu, Berry, & Kaplan, 1996; Sutton, 1996). In this section, we highlight some of these concerns and discuss them. The stages of change model has been proposed as one that isolates critical dimensions of the intentional behavior change process. In addition to its popularity with many addiction counselors and researchers, the model should prove to be useful for tracking and predicting change. Research findings should support the contentions of the model or at least be consistent with the constructs outlined by the model. Research can never prove a theory. However, research can weaken or disprove various aspects of a theory if the findings consistently contradict the basic assumptions of the model.

Stages or a Continuous Process?

Are there really stages of change, or is the process of change better viewed as a continuous one? Difficulties in classifying people into the specific stages (Joseph et al., 1999) and the criticism that stage models are not helpful for viewing process activities (Bandura, 1997) have produced challenges to the validity of the stage perspective. Critics question whether it is more useful to view the process of change as a single stream that flows around curves and barriers or whether it is better characterized as a series of stages that are distinct, sequential, and interconnected. The case against stages appears to be based on the view that the process of change must either be a multidimensional continuous one or one that has distinct stages. If this dualistic view of the process of change must be chosen, the multidimensional continuous view seems more appealing. However, according to the developers of the stages of change model, these two conceptualizations do not have to appear on opposite sides of the debate (Prochaska & DiClemente, 1998). Depending on the chosen definition of stages, the permeability of the boundaries between stages, and the breadth of the perspective taken, the process of human behavior change can be viewed as both—a continuous process with important discrete steps. A staircase is really a straight line from one floor to another. However, without the steps it would be difficult to negotiate the passage. A life span view of recovery from alcoholism, for example, can identify a course of change over time that for some clients looks like a steady stream of activity leading to successful problem resolution. In fact, the famous Jellinek U-shaped curve depicted the process of becoming addicted and recovering as a smooth curvilinear function, indicating that the individual descended into addiction, hit bottom, and then moved upward into recovery (DiClemente & Scott, 1997). However, the process does not appear to be linear or curvilinear.

That same life span view of addiction and recovery indicates that most individuals have followed problematic paths over many years and made multiple attempts to change before being successful (Vaillant, 1995). Individuals get stuck at certain points in this process of change and invest more time and energy in *not* changing or thinking about change than in activities that would promote change. Taking actions that result in relapse or maintenance represent important distinct steps in successful recovery. For some, the goal of recovery is elusive even with multiple attempts to change. For most, the process of change is filled with periods of movement as well as long periods of time spent maintaining the status quo of the habit. As we tie together the different events in a life of addiction and recovery, there seems to be both an ebb and a flow in the process of change and important, distinct tasks that mark the process. Continuous and discrete-stage perspectives on the process of change are not necessarily contradictory. In fact, they can be complementary (Prochaska & DiClemente, 1998).

The stages are described as a way of segmenting the process of change into useful but rather fluid states (DiClemente & Prochaska, 1998). Individuals can move forward and backward through the stages, and they can do so quickly. The critical defining feature of a stage seems to be whether there are important distinguishable tasks that need to be accomplished to achieve movement toward successful behavior change. However, these tasks do not appear to have the same characteristics from one stage to the next, as would be observed in developmental stage theories that mark the growth of an organism. Growth indicators like increases in height or the transition from caterpillar to butterfly have only a single direction and never proceed in opposite directions. Butterflies never become caterpillars, and people become taller until reaching full development. These developmental stages are unidirectional, discrete, self-contained states that are discontinuous. On the other hand, the stages of change model represents a series of tasks that need to be accomplished before the individual can move from one stage to the next stage. These tasks involve a number of dimensions (motivation, decision making, efficacy, coping activities) that have an ongoing influence on the change process, can be accomplished quickly or slowly, and can be done more or less completely. From this perspective, the quality and completeness of the execution of the stage-specific tasks would impact success in the subsequent stages of the process of change. These stages of change, therefore, seem to be more like the stage dimensions of personality development proposed by Erikson (1963). Erikson viewed the psychological growth and maturation of an individual as a series of bipolar tasks (trust versus mistrust) that build on one another, become salient at certain points in the development of the individual, and can be more or less resolved as the individual moves through life. If stages of change are envisioned more like Eriksonian stages, then the debate over a continuous versus a discrete-stage process seems less important. Both continuous processes and important discrete tasks appear to represent critical components of the process of change.

The research to date appears to support a process of change for substance abusers that has a series of steps or phases that require different strategies and address different issues. Processes of change, decision-making self-evaluations, and relevant efficacy evaluations vary significantly by stage of change (DiClemente & Prochaska, 1998; DiClemente, Prochaska, & Gibertini, 1985; DiClemente et al., 1991; Smith et al., 1991; Prochaska et al., 1991, 1992, 1994; Velasquez et al., 1999). There is also evidence that shifting process activity as one moves from contemplation and preparation to action is the more effective way to achieve successful smoking cessation (Perz et al., 1996). Movement through the process of change does not appear to be a case of doing more of the same thing, as would be expected in a purely continuous model, but instead a case of doing the right thing at the right time. The developers of the model have proposed that the research evidence of significant differences among individuals in the different stages of change on decisional balance, self-efficacy, and processes of change offer support for the importance of the discrete stage perspective. The interrelationship between the stages and these other critical dimensions of change are at the heart of the model. The fact that these differences between stages have been found with change across different types of behaviors (exercise adoption, modification of alcohol problems, smoking cessation, condom use) seems to offer significant support to that contention. However, it is also important to note that the proponents of the model have always looked across stages and created graphic representations of process activity, efficacy, and decisional considerations that are continuous and either linear or curvilinear in shape across the different stages (Prochaska et al., 1991). Pros and cons for change do seem to rise or fall across the stages in a curvilinear fashion (Prochaska et al., 1994). Self-efficacy appears to rise as individuals move from precontemplation through the stages to maintenance (DiClemente et al., 1985). Some processes appear to rise in early stages and then decline in occurrence during action and maintenance (Prochaska et al., 1991).

Relapse as an Event

It is also interesting to note how the proponents of the model have handled the issue of relapse. Initially relapse was viewed as a potential stage of change (Prochaska & DiClemente, 1982). However, as data on the processes of change used by relapsers became clearer, relapse appeared to be better categorized as an event rather than a stage of change (DiClemente & Prochaska, 1998). In fact, all relapsers can be categorized in terms of their current stage of change. Thus, it makes more sense to envision and classify individuals who recently relapsed as recycling through the earlier stages of precontemplation, contemplation, and preparation rather than being in a separate stage (Prochaska & DiClemente, 1984; DiClemente & Prochaska, 1998). There do appear to be important distinctions among the events that occur on the road to recovery before and after a relapse that have implications for moving through the stages of change. An unsuccessful attempt to quit the substance abuse can indicate that the individual is better prepared to make another attempt that may be more successful. Some definitions of the preparation stage include a recent quit attempt (DiClemente et al., 1991). Once again, this seems to indicate that stages are based on particular tasks that mark a continuous, albeit circuitous, route to recovery from substance abuse and dependence to sobriety and abstinence.

When Did the Preparation Stage Appear?

Another concern that critics have voiced about the stages of change model is that the stages simply represent labels that help clinicians classify clients but do not reflect detectable steps in the process of change that predict change (Davidson, 1992; Pierce et al., 1996). One part of this critique has already been answered above. Yet, there have been different stages proposed in earlier and later versions of the model. An early version has only precontemplation, contemplation, action, and maintenance stages. A preparation stage was added later (DiClemente et al., 1991). Some authors reporting on an early version of the model identify a determination stage (Miller & Rollnick, 1991). The proponents of the model claim that measuring the determination (early version) or preparation (later version) stage has been challenging, and therefore some versions of the model have included only four stages since these were the only ones that could be reliably measured (Prochaska & DiClemente,

1984). More current versions of the model have included a preparation stage (DiClemente & Prochaska, 1998).

The issue of assessment is a particularly complicated one, and we will examine it in detail later. However, it does seem to be reasonable that assessment and theory building be integrated. If a construct cannot be measured, it cannot be evaluated. One can hypothesize the existence of many different constructs, as the history of clinical psychology will attest. However, many of these constructs have not been able to be tested because they have not been operationalized (defined in a measurable way). The attempt to make assumptions and to revise the model based on empirical data appears to be a strength of the stages model rather than a weakness. Changing names and constructs do pose problems for those wanting to apply the model. However, the real test appears to be whether these stages can be identified, measured, and used in ways that are helpful and supported by research.

Prediction of Outcomes

Another concern is whether the stages are related to outcomes, as expected by the model. Although the data are not conclusive, there is a growing body of literature that appears to support the relationship of stages to important clinical outcomes. Although not supported in every study, stage status has been related to participation in program activities like reading self-help materials (DiClemente et al., 1991), attendance at treatment sessions (Smith, Subich, & Kolodner, 1995), and outcomes of interventions (DiClemente et al., 1991; Project MATCH Research Group, 1997a). Changes in stage from one time point to another (Carbonari et al., 1999) and increasing and decreasing levels of process of change activities by stage (Prochaska et al., 1991) also support the relationship of stage status with progress and the process of recovery. Stages and the related concept of readiness to change have been predictive of the amount and extent of change. In several studies stage-related status predicted attempts to change and successful outcomes (Carbonari & DiClemente, 2000; DiClemente et al., 1991; Tsoh, 1995; Project MATCH Research Group, 1997a, 1997b, 1998a).

In Project MATCH, a microanalysis of the influence of client readiness to change assessed as individuals entered outpatient treatment indicated that readiness predicted client evaluations of the quality of the therapeutic relationship, level of coping activities both during and at the end of treatment, and drinking quantity and frequency during posttreatment (DiClemente,

Carbonari, Zweben, et al., 2001; Connors et al., 2000). However, there was little support for a treatment-matching effect between baseline motivation and the Project MATCH motivational enhancement treatment (Project MATCH Research Group, 1997a, 1998a). Although there is intriguing support for the role of motivation and stages in the prediction of outcomes for substance abuse treatments, more research is needed. In addition, studies are needed that examine the interaction of stage status with a variety of other variables so that the joint and unique predictive ability of all these variables can be better understood. There is evidence that currently supports the predictive validity of the stages. However, it is far from conclusive or incontrovertible at the present time.

Labels—or Aids to Intervention?

The criticism that stages are simply labels would be justified if providers sought to identify precontemplators in order to deny them services or did not use these stages as a way to conceptualize what is going on for the client in that particular stage and how they can help him or her move to the next step. If stages were used simply as labels to stigmatize people (e.g., as hopeless precontemplators), they would be useless. This would be similar to viewing everyone not ready for action as in denial. However, these stages have spurred many clinicians to develop alternative strategies for welcoming precontemplators into treatment and addressing their needs specifically. Miller and Rollnick (1991) have outlined motivational interviewing procedures to address individuals in precontemplation and contemplation, in particular. Clinicians and researchers have come together to outline strategies and procedures to move individuals through each of the stages of change (Miller, 1999; Rollnick et al., 1999; Shaffer, 1992; Velasquez, Maurer, Crouch, & DiClemente, 2001). Programs have been developed to reach out proactively to precontemplators and to engage them in the process of change with good success (DiClemente & Prochaska, 1998; Velicer et al., 1993). In general, the stage construct does appear to have utility beyond mere categorization of individuals and has generated innovative approaches to treatment of substance abusers.

Measuring the Stages

Measurement of stages of change poses a particular problem for the practitioner and the researcher. How to assess the stage status of individuals with different substance abuse problems and in different types of programs has created significant frustration with the construct of stages (Carey, Purnine, Maisto, & Carey, 1999; Joseph et al., 1999). Multiple measures have been used, including categorical algorithms, ladders or rulers, grids, and multiple item, multiple subscale questionnaires like the URICA (McConnaughy et al., 1989), the SOCRATES (Miller & Tonigan, 1996), and readiness-to-change scales (Carbonari, DiClemente, & Zweben, 1994; DiClemente & Prochaska, 1998; Heather et al., 1993). The good news is that many different measures have been able to divide the population of changers into subgroups that make sense and are consistent with the idea of stages (Carney & Kivlahan, 1995; Isenhart, 1994; Willoughby & Edens, 1996). However, the bad news is that there is no single measure of stage status for all behaviors. It is also significant that the different measures do not always cross-classify individuals into the same stage of change (Belding, Iguchi, & Lamb, 1996; Carey, Purnine, Maisto, & Carey, 1999; Joseph et al., 1999; Rothfleisch, 1997). However, the importance of readiness to change is supported in many different studies (DeLeon et al., 1994; DiClemente, 1999b; Simpson & Joe, 1993).

The problems with assessing stage status appear to be related to four issues. First, the target goal of the behavior change often is poorly specified. Second, measures have been poorly constructed and inadequately evaluated. Third, measures must rely on self-report and the accuracy and honesty of the individual reporting his or her behavior and attitudes. Fourth, stage status is difficult to assess since it represents a mobile state and not a static trait.

There are several important dimensions that need to be addressed in accurately assessing stage status. These include having a clear behavioral target (abstinence or reduction), attitudes toward changing that behavior in the future (next 6 months or next month), accepted indicators of actual behavior change, and length of time the change has been sustained (DiClemente & Prochaska, 1998). However, the application is not a simple matter, particularly when the target behavior is complex and multifaceted or when there are multiple potential goals with regard to the target behavior. Reducing drinking and abstaining from drinking represent two different potential goals for an alcohol abuser. Stage status related to these two distinct goals could be very different. Some polydrug clients are prepared to take action with regard to one drug but not another, so a generic stage status related to illegal drugs would likely miss client readiness with one or the other drug. Specificity of behavior and of the change goal is critical for accurate assessment.

The multiple measures of stage status are a mixed blessing. The fact that multiple measures can be used successfully supports the notion that the process of change can be segmented, as well as the existence of some underlying idea, like stages of change. These assessments create ways to identify whether the individual is in earlier or later segments of the process of change. Some measures attempt to create stage subgroups; others are satisfied with simply identifying individuals who are more or less ready to change. However, using either continuous measures or stage-based classifications, individuals earlier in the process differ from individuals in later stages on measures of change process activity, decisional considerations, and self-efficacy. Although measuring these stages in different behaviors has proved challenging, different measures seem to have identified individuals at different points in the process of change with many addictive and other behaviors.

Research on the stages requires accurate assessment of where clients are in the process of change. That assessment is almost completely reliant on the self-report of the individual substance abuser. There are some biochemical assessments that can verify the self-report of abstinence from certain substances. Samples of blood, breath, saliva, urine, and even hair can be used to see whether an individual has used a particular substance within the immediate past day, week or, at best, month. These tests yield only an assessment of abstinence and typically cannot examine reduction in use, binge episodes, and other irregular patterns of use. So, even for the evaluation of action and maintenance stage status, the therapist must necessarily rely on the self-report of the substance abuser. And it is clear that reliable reporting of attitudes and behavior is even more critical to the assessment of earlier stages.

Although social pressure, situational demands, and self-deception can influence the self-reports of substance abusers, there is no reason to abandon self-report. The client's perspective is the most important one in the treatment process. The key objective is to create an environment where the client can report honestly and to ask questions that allow the client to characterize his or her attitudes and behaviors in ways that are comfortable. Asking a client who comes to treatment as a condition of parole whether he or she wants to stop using cocaine on the first day in the clinic is problematic. This would be particularly true if the client believed that saying yes was essential to entry into treatment. However, cigarette smoking evokes less concern, and most of the time asking a series of questions about current smoking and readiness to quit smoking yields a pretty good assessment of a smoker's stage of change (DiClemente &

Prochaska, 1998). However, there have been numerous problems with using a similar set of questions during intake to a drug abuse program (Rothfleisch, 1997; Belding et al., 1996). A less direct approach may be needed with other substance abuse behaviors. As described in the assessment chapter, the SOCRATES and versions of the URICA have been rather successful in assessing readiness to change and stage-related groups (DiClemente & Hughes, 1990; Carney & Kivlahan, 1995; Willoughby & Edens, 1996). In both of these assessments, clients are asked a series of questions representing a number of attitudes and views that they can endorse by using a range of responses and not simply yes or no. When given the opportunity to endorse a little or a lot, clients give a more accurate view of where they are in the process of change. However, there needs to be much additional research on how to evaluate stage status in different settings and with different substance abuse problems.

Some of the difficulty in assessing stage status is due to the nature of the stages of change. Stages represent the current state of the individual with respect to changing a single behavior. Stage status can persist for a long time or could change in a very short time. An individual who is in precontemplation about quitting smoking today could be in preparation or action tomorrow after learning about the death of his best friend from lung cancer. Assessing this moving target and then using that single intake assessment to predict change outcomes is problematic. It is all the more astounding that the stage variables have been very potent predictors in many studies despite all the problems described above. A measure should operationalize a construct in a satisfactory manner. However, no measure is ever a complete measure of a construct. There are multiple behavior-specific measures of the construct of self-efficacy, for example. Each measure is only an approximation of the efficacy construct applied to a particular behavior and behavioral goal. Similarly, multiple assessments of stages must be viewed as unique efforts at approximating the stage status of an individual.

Multiple Problems and a Common Process

One of the advantages for those who are using the stages of change model in treatment is that the process of change outlined in the model is assumed to be the same for substance abuse problems as well as other life problems. The model has been applied to changing many different behaviors, including positive health behaviors like exercise and cancer screening as well as problems such as medication compliance, anxiety and depression, and obesity (Beitman et al., 1994; Bowen & Trotter, 1995; Grimley, Riley, Bellis, & Prochaska, 1993; Marcus, Rossi, Selby, Niaura, & Abrams, 1992; McConnaughy et al., 1989). Stages and processes of change have been evaluated in a variety of these behaviors. The process appears to be similar across the various behaviors. Clinicians who use the model can think about the various problems that the substance abusing client has on entry to treatment in a similar way (DiClemente et al., 1992). Some clients are very ready to deal with one problem while being in early stages with regard to another problem. The ability to view the multiple problems of a client, be they various drugs of abuse or in other areas of life, in terms of a single change process appears to be an important advantage for the clinician.

Treatment of substance abuse has often been viewed as very different from treatment of mental health, relationships, adjustment, and physical health problems. In that way, substance abuse treatment has been isolated and "carved out" of traditional health care considerations. Although some critics view the breadth of application of the stages of change model to multiple problem areas to be a negative, substance abuse treatment providers can use this breadth of scope to assist them in dealing with the many other problems of the substance abuser. Moreover, the commonality of this process of change across different types of behaviors argues for substance abuse treatment to be included in the broad continuum of care that should be provided to individuals in the community rather than being an isolated treatment service (DiClemente, 1999a; McLellan, Arndt, Metzger, Woody, & O'Brien, 1993).

Adequacy of the Stages of Change Model

A final criticism of the stages of change model is that it focuses on individual change dimensions and has a limited perspective. Some critics argue that there exist other more comprehensive and explanatory theories, like Bandura's social cognitive theory (1986), that can explain change. The implication is that the stages of change model misses important dimensions and is not comprehensive.

There is a significant difference between a model and a theory. The architects of the stages of change model have focused the model on the process of intentional behavior change and claim that the model has a narrower focus than the more global theories of human functioning

(DiClemente & Prochaska, 1998; Joseph et al., 1999). Nonetheless, the stages do cover a considerable amount of ground, since the process of intentional behavior change is central in the life of the individual, with major implications for human growth and development.

The stages of change model has been applied to multiple types of behavior changes, from sunscreen use to cocaine addiction. There are few models that can be applied to such a variety of behaviors with such consistent results. However, the application of the model to these multiple behaviors is sometimes conducted without proper attention being paid to important differences among these behaviors. This fuels some of the criticism about the model reaching beyond its scope or appropriate applicability. It may also be true that some proponents appear to make claims for the model that encourage critics to compare the model to a more general theory of human functioning. The model should be judged in the context of the rather narrow focus of intentional behavior change (rather than all human functioning). In this context, the broad applicability to behavior change despite the clear differences among these behaviors (exercise, drinking, smoking, condom use) supports the construct validity of the stages and processes of change. Attempts to use this as a broad theory of human functioning or to compare it to such a theory are misguided.

FUTURE DIRECTIONS

Although there have been a substantial number of studies that have applied the stages of change model to substance abuse problems, there is much to learn about the stages and how the model can most productively be used in clinical practice. In this volume we have identified issues, strategies, and interventions that target individuals in the various stages of change. However, clinicians and researchers must continue to examine how to support movement through the stages more effectively and efficiently and to identify which techniques or strategies would be most successful with clients in these stages. In particular, we need to know how to get individuals moving who are stuck in the precontemplation and contemplation stages of change, understand the critical parameters of planning needed in the preparation stage, and evaluate the most effective ways to promote recycling. We also need to know more specifics about how the process of change works with different groups of individuals in recovery, such as those who only go to Alcoholics Anonymous (Snow,

Prochaska, & Rossi, 1994; DiClemente, 1993) and those who are dually diagnosed (Bellack & DiClemente, 1999; Velasquez et al., 1999). Another important challenge concerns the training of individuals to deliver appropriate interventions across the entire spectrum of the process of change.

Substance abusers as well as other types of changers take a long time to move through these stages of change once they have a well-established pattern of drug or alcohol dependence. Over a 6-month period without intervention, the majority of individuals in the earlier stages of change will remain in precontemplation or contemplation (Carbonari et al., 1999). Previous research has identified large numbers of contemplators who remain in contemplation for long periods of time and has labeled these individuals "chronic contemplators" (Prochaska et al., 1991). Encouraging movement out of these initial stages is not easy for "virgin quitters" as they move through the stages making a first attempt to stop drinking or drugging. However, once individuals have been through the cycle and failed, it can be even harder to get them to move through again. An important consideration is that the process of change occurs in the natural environment and not simply during treatment or intervention (DiClemente, 1999a). Most individuals who come into treatment, therefore, are not naive "change virgins" who have never tried to modify or stop their problematic substance use. Many have been through the cycle of change on their own several times before asking for help (DiClemente & Scott, 1997). Sometimes they expect treatment to make change happen with little effort on their part. At other times they need to be convinced that it would be worthwhile to leave precontemplation or contemplation again to make another attempt to solve the drug abuse problem. Getting individuals to move forward out of these stages is a significant challenge.

Several strategies have been identified that can be used as motivational enhancement strategies (Miller & Rollnick, 1991; Miller, 1999). However, continued thought and effort should be dedicated to researching and designing ways of specifically encouraging individuals to move out of precontemplation and contemplation. As the legal system becomes more aggressive in mandating drug and alcohol offenders to treatment, the need to develop strategies that engage the client in an intentional process of change during mandated interventions or an imposed suspension of the drug abuse behavior become more important. There is room for creativity and ingenuity on the part of the clinician and researcher alike to design and evaluate new interventions to help these early-stage individuals break the logjam and move forward in the process of change.

One of the important parts of preparing individuals for action is promoting and increasing commitment to action. The descriptions of the preparation stage detail both developing a change plan and increasing commitment as the two critical tasks to be accomplished during that stage. Clinicians are given little training in how to enhance commitment to follow through on an action plan. Albert Ellis and colleagues have written about defeating procrastination (Ellis & Dryden, 1987), which seems to be part of the problem. However, techniques and strategies that frankly address commitment enhancement are rare and not taught as part of substance abuse counseling programs. Goal setting, choice, and going public have all been identified as potential commitment enhancement tools (Miller, 1999). These and other similar techniques need to be evaluated in the context of preparation stage activity in order to see which are the most important. How to increase commitment effectively represents a significant challenge for the field.

Another important issue in the treatment of substance abuse involves the reality of relapse and how relapse impacts movement through the stages of change. The stages of change model has identified a recycling process in which relapse becomes an event that creates a cyclical movement back through the stages of change. However, how this occurs, what the critical dimensions of the recycling events are, and what interventions yield the most efficient recycling have not yet been established. Relapse appears to be a critical event in the process of recovery that influences how long recovery will take for any individual. It is an important learning experience that can encourage, discourage, or derail positive movement through the change process. Although there has been extensive research on relapse and relapse prevention (Marlatt & Gordon, 1985; Marlatt, 1996), knowledge about the event, its precipitants, and, most importantly, its role in the overall view of recovery is not well understood. Clinicians and researchers need to take a broader view of the process of recovery when dealing with clients or designing studies. Where the client has been in the process of change prior to entering treatment is as important as the specific goals of the client.

Relapse is not the only area where additional research is needed to assist clinicians in applying the stages and processes of change. Other critical areas need clarification and better understanding, including measuring the stages of change, the relationship of stage transitions to long-term outcomes, and how different treatments interact with the process of change.

As the chapter on assessment (Chapter 3) and our discussion on measurement have pointed out, there are significant problems in ascertaining exactly where an individual is in the process of change with many of the assessment instruments. Clinicians seem to have less of a problem identifying stage status when they can talk with an individual client openly and honestly and when they can access thoughts and feelings as well as watch his or her behavior over time. What seems to be needed are multiple indicators that would enable the clinician and researcher to pinpoint the stage status of an individual across several dimensions. In a recent book titled *Health Behavior Change*, Rollnick and colleagues (1999) discussed the importance of the change and the confidence to make the change as important and rather independent dimensions that can influence readiness to change. Decisional balance considerations or the relations between the pros and cons of change would be another possible indicator. Appropriate change process activity could also become a marker of stage status once we have some norms for individuals seeking treatment. In any case, there is a need for significant additional research in assessing the stages and the related constructs so that clinicians can better classify individuals along the steps in the process of change.

Another issue that needs much additional research involves the relationship between stage transitions and long-term outcomes. How important is the completion of stage-specific tasks to the overall achievement of successful maintenance? Is it better to have individuals make some half-hearted attempts to change or to have them wait and make only serious ones? How does external pressure to enter treatment affect the movement from one stage to the next for individuals in precontemplation versus contemplation? Is there an ideal amount of time that needs to be spent in a stage, or is it completely variable? Do individuals who are stuck in a particular stage for a long period of time fare better or worse in achieving their ultimate goal? Some of the most informative data we have about some of these issues come from following smokers over long periods of time. However, it is not clear if the patterns and process for smoking cessation are exactly the same as the ones for heroin, cocaine, or alcohol. There has not been enough research to make all the comparisons needed, and there is still much to learn about the process of recovery for smoking cessation as well as other drugs of abuse. Longitudinal research with large numbers of individuals is needed to answer these questions. Capturing this process in the natural environment is not an easy task. It is not easy to accumulate the numbers of individuals needed to have the power to be able to predict outcomes for each stage of change. With so many individuals being stuck in stages for long periods of time, it is difficult to capture enough changers at any one time to make certain predictions with very large numbers of research participants willing to participate over many years. Nevertheless, the need for such research to resolve some basic questions about the process of change for substance abusers is obvious.

Understanding this process of change is of paramount importance. However, it probably cannot be studied without examining the relationship between the process and the various treatments to which substance abusers are exposed. How treatment interacts with the process of change is another important avenue for continued research. At present, the evidence indicates that different types of treatments influence the process of change in similar ways (Prochaska, DiClemente, Velicer, & Rossi, 1993; DiClemente, Carbonari, Zweben, et al., 2001). In Project MATCH the three different treatments (cognitive-behavioral, motivational enhancement, and 12-step facilitation) resulted in very similar client process activity and equivalent levels of abstinence self-efficacy. Miller and Rollnick (1991) indicate that motivational interviewing is particularly important for individuals in early stages of change. However, research evidence for these claims needs to be gathered. A question remaining is whether we can find treatments that differentially impact processes of change so as to match clinical interventions to specific stages.

Finally, there are some interesting phenomena that can be explored using the stages of change perspective. Recent research on smoking cessation with pregnant women indicates that these women may temporarily stop rather than quit smoking during pregnancy (Stotts, DiClemente, Carbonari, & Mullen, 1996). Even after extensive periods of abstinence during pregnancy, women relapse at very high rates immediately postpartum. They seem to be suspending the behavior rather than changing it, and their attitudes toward postpartum smoking appear to be critical in predicting the return to smoking (Stotts, DiClemente, Carbonari, & Mullen, 2000). These findings lead to a broader discussion of imposed and extrinsically motivated change compared to intrinsic and chosen change (DiClemente, 1999b). With the increasing use of court-mandated treatment and efforts to provide treatment in prison settings, the issues of extrinsic and intrinsically motivations for change and how they interact with the process of change need an extensive examination and additional research.

A similar issue arises when discussing harm reduction strategies. Do harm reduction strategies interfere with successful movement through the process of change outlined in this volume? Harm reduction and recovery from substance abuse problems do not have to be at odds since the concerns that encourage individuals to take some harm reduction steps could also serve to tip the decisional balance toward action for a more complete change. However, whether each of the specific harm reduction strategies does or does not function as a facilitator of change, or at least does not prove to be a barrier to complete recovery, requires extensive research into how harm reduction affects the process of change.

CONCLUSION

This volume offers clinicians a view of treatment that is informed by the stages of change model. The recommendations are based on our view of the current literature and the clinical applications of this model. Since researchers and practitioners continue to apply this model to different populations and problems and to refine the constructs, clinical application continues to be a work in progress. Additional knowledge and insights will undoubtedly emerge as this work progresses. We hope we have provided the clinician some new strategies and views with which to assist those struggling with substance abuse problems to move forward on the road to recovery.

SUMMARY

• The stages of change model focuses on the identification of important components in the process of intentional behavior change. The stages highlight the critical issues of denial, decision making, anticipation, action, relapse, and maintenance for specific behavioral problems.

• A significant contribution of the model is the identification of different tasks and challenges faced by the client and the therapist at different points in the process of changing addictive behaviors.

• There is debate in the literature on some aspects of the stages of change model. One particular issue of note is whether the process of change is most productively viewed as involving stages of change or as a continuous process. It is argued here that the process of change for substance abusers involves a series of stages or phases that require different strategies and address different issues.

- While much has been written about the application of the stages of change model to substance abuse problems, there is more to be learned about the stages and how the model can be most productively used in clinical practice. Additional knowledge and insights will undoubtedly emerge as researchers and practitioners continue to apply the model to different populations and problems.

REFERENCES

Addiction Research Foundation. (1993). *Directory of client outcome measures for addictions treatment programs.* Toronto: Author.

Addington, J., el-Guebaly, N., Duchak, V., & Hodgins, D. (1999). Using measures of readiness to change in individuals with schizophrenia. *American Journal of Drug and Alcohol Abuse, 25,* 151–161.

Agency for Health Care Policy and Research. (1996). *Clinical practice guideline for smoking cessation.* AHCPR Guideline Number 18. Washington, DC: Author.

Ahijevych, K., & Wewers, M. E. (1992). Processes of change across five stages of smoking cessation. *Addictive Behaviors, 17,* 17–25.

Ahles, T. A., Schlundt, D. G., Prue, D. M., & Rychtarik, R. G. (1983). Impact of aftercare arrangements on the maintenance of treatment success in abusive drinkers. *Addictive Behaviors, 8,* 53–58.

Allan, C. A., & Cooke, D. J. (1985). Stressful life events and alcohol misuse in women: A critical review. *Journal of Studies on Alcohol, 46,* 147–152.

Allen, J. C., & Columbus, M. (Eds.). (1995). *Assessing alcohol problems.* Rockville, MD: National Institute on Alcohol Abuse and Alcoholism.

Allen, K. (1994). Development of an instrument to identify barriers to treatment for addicted women, from their perspective. *International Journal of the Addictions, 29,* 429–444.

Allsop, S., & Saunders, B. (1991). Reinforcing robust resolutions: Motivation in relapse prevention with severely dependent problem drinkers. In W. R. Miller & S. Rollnick (Eds.), *Motivational interviewing: Preparing people to change addictive behavior* (pp. 236–247). New York: Guilford Press.

Alterman, A. I., Brown, L. S., Zaballero, A., & McKay, J. R. (1994). Interviewer severity

239

ratings and composite scores of the ASI: A further look. *Drug and Alcohol Dependence, 34*, 201–209.

American Psychiatric Association. (1994). *Diagnostic and statistical manual of mental disorders* (4th ed.). Washington, DC: Author.

Amrod, J. (1997). Effect of motivational enhancement therapy and coping skills training on the self-efficacy and motivation of incarcerated male alcohol abusers. *Dissertation Abstracts International, 57*, 5904-B–5905-B.

Anderson, C. M., & Stewart, S. (1983). *Mastering resistance: A practical guide to family therapy.* New York: Guilford Press.

Anderson, D. J. (1981). *The psychopathology of denial.* Minneapolis: Hazelden.

Anker, A. L., & Crowley, T. J. (1982). Use of contingency contracts in specialty clinics for cocaine abuse. In L. S. Harris (Ed.), *Problems of drug dependence, 1981* (pp. 452–459). Washington, DC: National Institute on Drug Abuse.

Annis, H. M. (1982a). *Inventory of Drinking Situations.* Toronto: Addiction Research Foundation.

Annis, H. M. (1982b). *Situational Confidence Questionnaire.* Toronto: Addiction Research Foundation.

Annis, H. M. (1986). A relapse prevention model for treatment of alcoholics. In W. R. Miller & N. Heather (Eds.), *Treating addictive behaviors* (pp. 407–433). New York: Plenum Press.

Annis, H. M. (1987). *Situational Confidence Questionnaire (SCQ-39).* Toronto: Addiction Research Foundation.

Annis, H. M., & Davis, C. S. (1988). Self-efficacy and the prevention of alcoholic relapse: Initial findings from a treatment trial. In T. B. Baker & D. S. Cannon (Eds.), *Assessment and treatment of addictive disorders.* New York: Praeger.

Annis, H. M., & Davis, C. S. (1991). Relapse prevention. *Alcohol Health and Research World, 15*, 204–212.

Annis, H. M., & Graham, J. M. (1988). *Situational Confidence Questionnaire (SCQ-39) user's guide.* Toronto: Addiction Research Foundation.

Annis, H. M., & Graham, J. M. (1995). Profile types on the Inventory of Drinking Situations: Implications for relapse prevention counseling. *Psychology of Addictive Behaviors, 9*, 176–182.

Annis, H. M., Graham, J. M., & Davis, C. S. (1987). *Inventory of Drinking Situations (IDS) user's guide.* Toronto: Addiction Research Foundation.

Annis, H. M., & Martin, G. (1985). *Drug-Taking Confidence Questionnaire.* Toronto: Addiction Research Foundation.

Annis, H. M., & Martin, G. (1993a). *The Inventory of Drug-Taking Situations.* Toronto: Addiction Research Foundation.

Annis, H. M., & Martin, G. (1993b). *The Drug-Taking Confidence Questionnaire.* Toronto: Addiction Research Foundation.

Annis, H. M., & Ogborne, A. C. (1983). *The temporal stability of alcoholism treatment outcome results.* Unpublished manuscript, Addiction Research Foundation.

Annis, H. M., Schober, R., & Kelly, E. (1996). Matching addiction outpatient counseling to client readiness for change: The role of structured relapse prevention counseling. *Experimental and Clinical Psychopharmacology, 4*, 37–45.

Anton, R. F., Litten, R. Z., & Allen, J. P. (1995). Biological assessment of alcohol consumption. In J. P. Allen & M. Columbus (Eds.), *Assessing alcohol problems* (pp. 31–40). Rockville, MD: National Institute on Alcohol Abuse and Alcoholism.

Armor, D., Polich, J., & Stambul, H. (1978). *Alcoholism and treatment.* New York: Wiley.

Azrin, N. H. (1976). Improvements in the community-reinforcement approach to alcoholism. *Behaviour Research and Therapy, 14,* 339–348.

Babor, T. F. (1993). Alcohol and drug use history, patterns, and problems. In B. J. Rounsaville, F. M. Tims, A. M. Horton, & B. J. Sowder (Eds.), *Diagnostic source book on drug abuse research and treatment* (pp. 19–34). Bethesda, MD: National Institute on Drug Abuse.

Babor, T. F., Kranzler, H. R., & Lauerman, R. J. (1989). Early detection of harmful alcohol consumption: Comparison of clinical, laboratory, and self-report screening procedures. *Addictive Behaviors, 14,* 139–157.

Baily, S. (1990). Women with alcohol problems: A psychosocial perspective. *Drug and Alcohol Review, 9,* 125–131.

Balgopal, P. R., & Hull, R. F. (1973). Keeping secrets: Group resistance for patients and therapists. *Psychotherapy: Theory, Research, and Practice, 10,* 334–336.

Bandura, A. (1977). Self-efficacy: Toward a unifying theory of behavioral change. *Psychological Review, 84,* 191–215.

Bandura, A. (1986). *Social foundations of thought and action: A social cognitive theory.* Englewood Cliffs, NJ: Prentice-Hall.

Bandura, A. (1997). The anatomy of stages of change [Editorial]. *American Journal of Health Promotion, 12,* 8–10.

Barber, J. G., & Gilbertson, R. (1997). Unilateral interventions for women living with heavy drinkers. *Social Work, 42,* 69–78.

Barber, W. S., & O'Brien, C. P. (1999) Pharmacotherapies. In B. S. McCrady & E. E. Epstein (Eds.), *Addiction: A comprehensive guidebook* (pp. 347–369). New York: Oxford University Press.

Barrie, K. (1991). Motivational counseling in groups. In R. Davidson, S. Rollnick, & I. MacEwan (Eds.), *Counseling problem drinkers* (pp. 115–131). London: Tavistock/Routledge.

Beckman, L. J. (1984a). Treatment needs of women alcoholics. *Alcoholism Treatment Quarterly, 1,* 101–114.

Beckman, L. J. (1984b). Analysis of the suitability of alcohol treatment resources for women. *Substance and Alcohol Actions/Misuse, 5,* 21–27.

Beckman, L. J., & Amaro, H. (1986). Personal and social difficulties faced by women and men entering alcoholism treatment. *Journal of Studies on Alcohol, 47,* 135–145.

Beitman, B. D., Beck, N. C., Deuser, W., Carter, C., Davidson, J., & Maddock, R. (1994). Patient stages of change predicts outcome in a panic disorder medication trial. *Anxiety, 1,* 64–69.

Belding, M., Iguchi, M., & Lamb, R. J. (1996). Stages of change in methadone maintenance: Assessing the convergent validity of two measures. *Psychology of Addictive Behaviors, 10,* 157–166.

Belding, M. A., Iguchi, M. Y., & Lamb, R. J. (1997). Stages and processes of change as predictors of drug use among methadone maintenance patients. *Experimental and Clinical Psychopharmacology, 5,* 65–73.

Belding, M., Iguchi, M., Lamb, R. J., Lakin, M., & Terry, R. (1995). Stages and processes of change among polydrug users in methadone maintenance treatment. *Drug and Alcohol Dependence, 30*, 45–53.

Bellack, A. S., & DiClemente, C. C. (1999). Treating substance abuse among patients with schizophrenia. *Psychiatric Services, 50*, 75–80.

Bennett, L. W. (1995). Substance abuse and the domestic assault of women. *Social Work, 40*, 760–771.

Berg, I. K., & Miller, S. D. (1992). *Working with the problem drinker: A solution-focused approach.* New York: Norton.

Beutler, L. E., & Clarkin, J. F. (1990). *Systematic treatment selection.* New York: Brunner/Mazel.

Bien, T., Miller, W., & Boroughs, J. (1993). Motivational interviewing with alcohol outpatients. *Behavioral and Cognitive Psychotherapy, 21*, 347–356.

Bierut, L. J., Dinwiddie, S. H., Begleiter, H., Crowe, R. R., Hesselbrock, V., Nurnberger, J. I., Jr., Porjesz, B., Schuckit, M. A., & Reich, T. (1998). Familial transmission of substance dependence: Alcohol, marijuana, cocaine, and habitual smoking. *Archives of General Psychiatry, 55*, 982–988.

Birke, S. A., Edelmann, R. J., & Davis, P. E. (1990). An analysis of the abstinence violation effect in a sample of illicit drug users. *British Journal of Addiction, 85*, 1299–1307.

Bland, R. C., Newman, S. C., & Orn, H. (1997). Help-seeking for psychiatric disorders. *Canadian Journal of Psychiatry, 42*, 935–942.

Booth, P. G., Dale, B., & Ansari, J. (1984). Problem drinkers' goal choice and treatment outcome: A preliminary study. *Addictive Behaviors, 9*, 357–364.

Bowen, A., & Trotter, R. (1995). HIV risk in intravenous drug users and crack cocaine smokers: Predicting stage of change for condom use. *Journal of Consulting and Clinical Psychology, 63*, 238–248.

Bradizza, C. M., & Stasiewicz, P. R. (1997). Integrating substance abuse treatment for the seriously mentally ill into inpatient psychiatric treatment. *Journal of Substance Abuse Treatment, 14*, 103.

Bradizza, C. M., Stasiewicz, P. R., & Carey, K. B. (1998). High-risk alcohol and drug use situations among seriously mentally ill inpatients: A preliminary investigation. *Addictive Behavior, 23*, 555–560.

Bradley, K. A., Boyd-Wickizer, J., Powell, S. H., & Burman, M. L. (1998). Alcohol screening questionnaires in women: A critical review. *Journal of the American Medical Association, 280*, 166–171.

Brady, K. T., & Randall, C. L. (1999). Gender differences in substance use disorders. *Psychiatric Clinics of North America, 22*, 241–252.

Brooke, D., Fudala, P. J., & Johnson, R. E. (1992). Weighing up the pros and cons: Help-seeking by drug misusers in Baltimore, USA. *Drug and Alcohol Dependence, 31*, 37–43.

Brown, S., & Yalom, I. (1977). Interactional group therapy with alcoholic patients. *Journal of Studies on Alcohol, 38*, 426–456.

Brownell, K. D., Marlatt, G. A., Lichtenstein, E., & Wilson, G. T. (1986). Understanding and preventing relapse. *American Psychologist, 41*, 765–782.

Bucholz, K. K., Homan, S. M., & Helzer, J. E. (1992). When do alcoholics first discuss drinking problems? *Journal of Studies on Alcohol, 53*, 582–589.

Burling, T. A., Reilly, P. M., Molzen, J. O., & Ziff, D. C. (1989). Self-efficacy and relapse among inpatient drug and alcohol abusers: A predictor of outcome. *Journal of Studies on Alcohol, 6,* 354–360.

Cannon, D. S., Leeka, J. K., Patterson, E. T., & Baker, T. B. (1990). Principal components analysis of the Inventory of Drinking Situations: Empirical categories of drinking by alcoholics. *Addictive Behavior, 15,* 265–269.

Carbonari, J. C., & DiClemente, C. C. (2000). Using transtheoretical model profiles to differentiate levels of alcohol abstinence success. *Journal of Consulting and Clinical Psychology, 68,* 810–817.

Carbonari, J. P., DiClemente, C. C., Addy, R., & Pollack, K. (1996). *Alternate short forms of the readiness to change scale.* Paper presented at the Fourth International Congress on Behavioral Medicine, Washington, DC.

Carbonari, J. P., DiClemente, C. C., & Sewell, K. B. (1999). Stage transitions and the transtheoretical "stages of change" model of smoking cessation. *Swiss Journal of Psychology, 58,* 134–144.

Carbonari, J., DiClemente, C., & Zweben, A. (November 1994). A readiness to change scale: Its development, validation and usefulness. In C. C. DiClemente (Chair), *Assessing critical dimensions for alcoholism treatment.* Symposium presented at the annual meeting of the Association for Advancement of Behavior Therapy, San Diego.

Carey, K. B. (1996). Substance use reduction in the context of outpatient psychiatric treatment: A collaborative, motivational, harm reduction approach. *Community Mental Health Journal, 32,* 291–306.

Carey, K. B., & Carey, M. P. (1995). Reasons for drinking among psychiatric outpatients: Relationship to drinking patterns. *Psychology of Addictive Behaviors, 9,* 251–257.

Carey, K. B., Purnine, D. M., Maisto, S. A., & Carey, M. P. (1999). Assessing readiness to change substance abuse: A critical review of instruments. *Clinical Psychology: Science and Practice, 6,* 245–266.

Carey, K. B., Purnine, D. M., Maisto, S. A., Carey, M. P., & Barnes, K. L. (1999). Decisional balance regarding substance use among persons with schizophrenia. *Community Mental Health Journal, 35,* 289–299.

Carney, M. M., & Kivlahan, D. R. (1995). Motivational subtypes among veterans seeking substance abuse treatment: Profiles based on stages of change. *Psychology of Addictive Behaviors, 9,* 135–142.

Carroll, K. M. (1996a). Integrating psychotherapy and pharmacotherapy in substance abuse treatment. In F. Rotgers, D. S. Keller, & J. Morgenstern (Eds.), *Treating substance abuse: Theory and technique* (pp. 286–318). New York: Guilford Press.

Carroll, K. M. (1996b). Relapse prevention as a psychosocial treatment: A review of controlled clinical trials. *Experimental and Clinical Psychopharmacology, 4,* 46–54.

Carroll, K. M. (1999). Behavioral and cognitive behavioral treatments. In B. S. McCrady & E. E. Epstein (Eds.), *Addiction: A comprehensive guidebook* (pp. 250–267). New York: Oxford University Press.

Cartwright, A. (1987). Group work with substance abusers: Basic issues and future research. *British Journal of Addiction, 82,* 951–953.

Cavaiola, A. A. (1984). Resistance issues in the treatment of the DWI offender. *Alcoholism Treatment Quarterly, 1,* 87–100.

Cermak, T. L. (1989). Al-Anon and recovery. In M. Galanter (Ed.), *Recent developments in alcoholism* (Vol. 7, pp. 91–104). New York: Plenum Press.

Chafetz, M. E. (1970). Practical and theoretical considerations in the psychotherapy of alcoholism. In M. E. Chafetz, H. T. Blane, & M. J. Hill (Eds.), *Frontiers of alcoholism* (pp. 6–15). New York: Science House.

Chaney, E. F. (1989). Social skills training. In R. K. Hester & W. R. Miller (Eds.), *Handbook of alcoholism treatment approaches* (pp. 206–221). New York: Pergamon Press.

Chang, G., Behr, H., Goetz, M. A., Hiley, A., & Bigby, J. (1997). Women and alcohol abuse in primary care: Identification and intervention. *American Journal on Addictions, 6,* 183–192.

Chassin, L., Curran, P. J., Hussong, A. M., & Colder, C. R. (1996). The relation of parent alcoholism to adolescent substance use: A longitudinal follow-up study. *Journal of Abnormal Psychology, 105,* 70–80.

Chessick, R. D. (1974). *Technique and practice of intensive psychotherapy.* New York: Jason Aronson.

Cialdini, R. B. (1988). *Influence: Science and practice* (2nd ed.). Glenview, IL: Scott Foresman & Company.

Connors, G. J. (1995). Screening for alcohol problems. In J. A. Allen & M. Columbus (Eds.), *Assessing alcohol problems* (pp. 17–29). Rockville, MD: National Institute on Alcohol Abuse and Alcoholism.

Connors, G. J., Carroll, K. M., DiClemente, C. C., Longabaugh, R., & Donovan, D. M. (1997). The therapeutic alliance and its relationship to alcoholism treatment participation and outcome. *Journal of Consulting and Clinical Psychology, 65,* 588–598.

Connors, G. J., DiClemente, C. C., Dermen, K. H., Kadden, R., Carroll, K. M., & Frone, M. R. (2000). Predicting the therapeutic alliance in alcoholism treatment. *Journal of Studies on Alcohol, 61,* 139–149.

Connors, G. J., Maisto, S. A., & Donovan, D. M. (1996). Conceptualizations of relapse: A summary of psychological and psychobiological models. *Addiction, 91*(Suppl.), 5–13.

Connors, G. J., Maisto, S. A., & Zywiak, W. H. (1996). Understanding relapse in the broader context of posttreatment functioning. *Addiction, 91*(Suppl.), 173–189.

Connors, G. J., Maisto, S. A., & Zywiak, W. H. (1998). Male and female alcoholics' attributions regarding the onset and termination of relapses and the maintenance of abstinence. *Journal of Substance Abuse, 10,* 27–42.

Cook, C. A. L., Booth, B. M., Blow, F. C., Gosineni, A., & Bunn, J. Y. (1992). Alcoholism treatment, severity of alcohol-related medical complications, and health services utilization. *Journal of Mental Health Administration, 19,* 31–40.

Copeland, J., & Hall, W. (1992). A comparison of women seeking drug and alcohol treatment in a specialist women's and two traditional mixed-sex treatment services. *British Journal of Addictions, 87,* 1293–1302.

Copeland, J., Hall, W., Didcott, P., & Biggs, V. (1993). A comparison of a specialist women's alcohol and other drug treatment service with two traditional mixed-sex services: Client characteristics and treatment outcome. *Drug and Alcohol Dependence, 32,* 81–92.

Costantini, M. F., Wermuth, L., Sorensen, J. L., & Lyons, J. S. (1992). Family functioning as a predictor of progress in substance abuse treatment. *Journal of Substance Abuse, 9,* 331–335.

Craighead, W. E., Craighead, L. W., & Ilardi, S. S. (1995). Behavior therapies in historical perspective. In B. Bongar & L. E. Beutler (Eds.), *Comprehensive textbook of psychotherapy* (pp. 64–83). New York: Oxford University Press.

Crits-Christoph, P., Siqueland, L., Blaine, J., Frank, A., Luborsky, L., Onken, L. S., Muenz, L. R., Thase, M. E., Weiss, R. D., Gastfriend, D. R., Woody, G. E., Barber, J. P., Butler, S. F., Daley, D., Salloum, I., Bishop, S., Najavits, L. M., Lis, J., Mercer, D., Griffin, M. L., Moras, K., & Beck, A. T. (1999). Psychosocial treatments for cocaine dependence: National Institute on Drug Abuse Collaborative Cocaine Treatment Study. *Archives of General Psychiatry, 57*, 493–502.

Cummings, C., Gordon, J. R., & Marlatt, G. A. (1980). Relapse: Prevention and prediction. In W. R. Miller (Ed.), *The addictive behaviors* (pp. 291–321). New York: Pergamon Press.

Cunningham, J. A., Sobell, L. C., Gavin, D. R., Sobell, M. B., & Breslin, F. C. (1997). Assessing motivation for change: Preliminary development and evaluation of a scale measuring the costs and benefits of changing alcohol or drug use. *Psychology of Addictive Behaviors, 11*, 107–114.

Cunningham, J. A., Sobell, L. C., Sobell, M. B., Argawal, S., & Toneatto, T. (1993). Barriers to treatment: Why alcohol and drug abusers delay or never seek treatment. *Addictive Behaviors, 18*, 347–353.

Cunningham, J. A., Sobell, L. C., Sobell, M. B., & Gaskin, J. (1994). Alcohol and drug abusers' reasons for seeking treatment. *Addictive Behaviors, 19*, 691–696.

Cunningham, J. A., Sobell, M. B., Sobell, L. C., Gavin, D. R., & Annis, H. (1995). Heavy drinking and negative affective situations in a general population and treatment sample: Alternative explanations. *Psychology of Addictive Behaviors, 9*, 123–127.

Cyr, M. G., & Wartman, S. A. (1988). The effectiveness of routine screening questions in the detection of alcoholism. *Journal of the American Medical Association, 259*, 51–54.

Daley, D. C., & Salloum, I. (1999). Relapse prevention. In P. J. Ott, R. E. Tarter, & R. T. Ammerman (Eds.), *Sourcebook on substance abuse: Etiology, epidemiology, assessment, and treatment* (pp. 255–263). Boston: Allyn & Bacon.

Daley, D. C., & Zuckoff, A. (1998). Improving compliance with the initial outpatient session among discharged inpatient dual diagnosis clients. *Social Work, 43*, 470–473.

Daniels, J. W. (1998). *Coping with the health threat of smoking: An analysis of the precontemplation stage of smoking cessation.* Doctoral dissertation, University of Maryland, Baltimore County.

Davidson, R. (1992). Prochaska & DiClemente's model of change: A case study? *British Journal of Addictions, 87*, 821–822.

DeAngelis, G. G. (1971). The role of urine testing in heroin treatment programs. *Journal of Psychedelic Drugs, 4*, 186–197.

DeLeon, G., Melnick, G., Kressel, D., & Jainchill, N. (1994). Circumstances, motivation, readiness and suitability (The CMRS scales): Predicting retention in therapeutic community treatment. *American Journal of Drug and Alcohol Abuse, 20*, 101–106.

DiClemente, C. C. (1991). Motivational interviewing and the stages of change. In W. R. Miller & S. Rollnick (Eds.), *Motivational interviewing: Preparing people to change addictive behavior* (pp. 191–202). New York: Guilford Press.

DiClemente, C. C. (1993) Alcoholics Anonymous and the structure of change. In B. S. McCrady & W. R. Miller (Eds.), *Research on Alcoholics Anonymous: Opportunities and alternatives* (pp. 79–97). New Brunswick, NJ: Rutgers Center of Alcohol Studies.

DiClemente, C. C. (1999a). Prevention and harm reduction for chemical dependency: A process perspective. *Clinical Psychology Review, 19,* 473–486.

DiClemente, C. C. (1999b). Motivation for change: Implications for substance abuse. *Psychological Science, 10,* 209–213.

DiClemente, C. C., Carbonari, J. P., Daniels, J., Donovan, D. M., Bellino, L. E., & Neavins, T. M. (2001). Self-efficacy as a matching hypothesis: Causal chain analysis. In R. Longabaugh & P. W. Wirth (Eds.), *Project MATCH: A priori matching hypotheses, results, and mediating mechanisms* (National Institute on Alcohol Abuse and Alcoholism Project MATCH Monograph Series, Vol. 8, pp. 251–269). Rockville, MD: National Institute on Alcohol Abuse and Alcoholism.

DiClemente, C. C., Carbonari, J. P., Montgomery, R. P. G., & Hughes, S. O. (1994). The Alcohol Abstinence Self-Efficacy Scale. *Journal of Studies on Alcohol, 55,* 141–148.

DiClemente, C. C., Carbonari, J. P., & Velasquez, M. M. (1992). Alcoholism treatment mismatching from a process of change perspective. In R. R. Watson (Ed.), *Treatment of drug and alcohol abuse* (pp. 115–142). Totowa, NJ: Humana Press.

DiClemente, C. C., Carbonari, J., Zweben, A., Morrel, T., & Lee., R. E. (2001). Motivational hypothesis causal chain analysis. In R. Longabaugh & P. W. Wirtz (Eds.), *Project MATCH: A priori matching hypotheses, results, and mediating mechanisms* (National Institute on Alcohol Abuse and Alcoholism Project MATCH Monograph Series, Vol. 8, pp. 218–234). Rockville, MD: National Institute on Alcohol Abuse and Alcoholism.

DiClemente, C. C., Gordon, J. R., & Gibertini, M. (1983). *Self-efficacy and determinants of relapse in alcoholism treatment.* Paper presented at the annual convention of the American Psychological Association, Anaheim, CA.

DiClemente, C. C., & Hughes, S. O. (1990). Stages of change profiles in outpatient alcoholism treatment. *Journal of Substance Abuse, 2,* 217–235.

DiClemente, C. C., & Prochaska, J. O. (1982). Self-change and therapy change of smoking behavior: A comparison of processes of change in cessation and maintenance. *Addictive Behaviors, 7,* 133–142.

DiClemente, C. C., & Prochaska, J. O. (1985). Processes and stages of change: Coping and competence in smoking behavior change. In S. Shiffman & T. A. Wills (Eds.), *Coping and substance abuse* (pp. 319–342). New York: Academic Press.

DiClemente, C. C., & Prochaska, J. O. (1998). Toward a comprehensive, transtheoretical model of change: Stages of change and addictive behaviors. In W. R. Miller & N. Heather (Eds.), *Treating addictive behaviors* (2nd ed., pp. 3–24). New York: Plenum Press.

DiClemente, C. C., Prochaska, J. O., Fairhurst, S. K., Velicer, W. F., Velasquez, M. M., & Rossi, J. S. (1991). The process of smoking cessation: An analysis of precontemplation, contemplation, and preparation stages of change. *Journal of Consulting and Clinical Psychology, 59,* 295–304.

DiClemente, C. C., Prochaska, J. O., & Gibertini, M. (1985). Self-efficacy and the stages of self-change smoking. *Cognitive Therapy and Research, 9,* 181–200.

DiClemente, C. C., & Scott, C. W. (1997). Stages of change: Interactions with treatment compliance and involvement. In L. S. Onken, J. D. Blaine, & J. J. Boren (Eds.), *Beyond the therapeutic alliance: Keeping the drug-dependent individual in treatment* (National Institute on Drug Abuse Research Monograph No. 165, pp. 131–156). Rockville, MD: National Institute on Drug Abuse.

Diesenhaus, H. I. (1982). Current trends in treatment programming for problem drinkers and alcoholics. In J. de Luca (Ed.), *Prevention, intervention, and treatments: Concerns and models* (pp. 219–290). Washington, DC: U.S. Government Printing Office.

Donovan, D. M. (1988). Assessment of addictive behaviors: Implications of an emerging biopsychosocial model. In D. M. Donovan & G. A. Marlatt (Eds.), *Assessment of addictive behaviors* (pp. 3–48). New York: Guilford Press.

Donovan, D. M. (1995). Assessments to aid in the treatment planning process. In J. P. Allen & M. Columbus (Eds.), *Assessing alcohol problems* (pp. 75–122). Rockville, MD: National Institute on Alcohol Abuse and Alcoholism.

Donovan, D. M. (1998). Continuing care: Promoting the maintenance of change. In W. R. Miller & N. Heather (Eds.), *Treating addictive behaviors* (2nd ed., pp. 317–336). New York: Plenum Press.

Donovan, D. M. (1999). Assessment strategies and measures in addictive behaviors. In B. S. McCrady & E. E. Epstein (Eds.), *Addiction: A comprehensive guidebook* (pp. 187–215). New York: Oxford University Press.

Donovan, D. M., & Chaney, E. F. (1985). Alcoholic relapse prevention and intervention: Models and methods. In G. A. Marlatt & J. R. Gordon (Eds.), *Relapse prevention* (pp. 351–416). New York: Guilford Press.

Donovan, D. M., & Marlatt, G. A. (Eds.). (1988). *Assessment of addictive behaviors.* New York: Guilford Press.

Donovan, D. M., & Rosengren, D. B. (1999). Motivation for behavior change and treatment among substance abusers. In J. A. Tucker, D. M. Donovan, & G. A. Marlatt (Eds.), *Changing addictive behavior: Bridging clinical and public health strategies* (pp. 127–159). New York: Guilford Press.

Drake, R. E., McLaughlin, P., Pepper, B., & Minkoff, K. (1991). Dual diagnosis of major mental illness and substance disorder: An overview. *New Directions in Mental Health Services, 50,* 3–12.

Drake, R. E., Mercer-McFadden, C., Mueser, K. T., McHugo, G. L., & Bond, G. R. (1998). Review of integrated mental health and substance abuse treatment for patients with dual disorders. *Schizophrenia Bulletin, 24,* 589–608.

Drake, R. E., & Noordsy, D. L. (1997). Treatment of comorbid disorders with a case manager approach. In N. S. Miller (Ed.), *Principles and practice of addictions in psychiatry* (pp. 221–228). Philadelphia: Saunders.

DuPont, R. L., & McGovern, J. P. (1996). Co-dependence. *The Hatherleigh guide to issues in modern therapy* (pp. 69–91). New York: Hatherleigh Press.

Egertson, J. A., Fox, D. M., & Leshner, A. I. (Eds.) (1997). *Treating drug abusers effectively.* Malden, MA: Blackwell.

Ehrman, R. N., & Robins, S. J. (1994). Reliability and validity of 6 month timeline reports of cocaine and heroin use in a methadone population. *Journal of Consulting and Clinical Psychology, 6,* 843–850.

Elkin, I, Shea, M. T., Watkins, J. T., Imber, S. D., Sotsky, S. M., Collins, J. F., Glass, D. R., Pilkinis, P. A., Leber, W. R., Docherty, J. P., Fiester, S. J., & Parloff, M. B. (1989). National Institute of Mental Health Treatment of Depression Collaborative Research Program: General effectiveness of treatments. *Archives of General Psychiatry, 46,* 971–982.

Ellis, A. (1983a). Rational-emotive therapy (RET) approaches to overcoming resistance: I. Common forms of resistance. *British Journal of Cognitive Psychotherapy, 1,* 28–38.

Ellis, A. (1983b). Rational-emotive therapy (RET) approaches to overcoming resistance: II. How RET disputes clients' irrational, resistance-creating beliefs. *British Journal of Cognitive Psychotherapy, 1,* 1–16.

Ellis, A. (1984). Rational-emotive therapy (RET) approaches to overcoming resistance: III. Using emotive and behavioral techniques of overcoming resistance. *British Journal of Cognitive Psychotherapy, 2,* 11–26.

Ellis, A. (1985). Approaches to overcoming resistance: IV. Handling special kinds of clients. *British Journal of Cognitive Psychotherapy, 1,* 26–42.

Ellis, A., & Dryden, W. (1987). *The practice of rational-emotive therapy.* New York: Springer.

Ellis, A., McInerney, J. F., DiGiuseppe, R. (1988). *Rational-emotive therapy with alcoholics and substance abusers.* Elmsford, NY: Pergamon.

Ends, E. J., & Page, C. W. (1957). A study of three types of group psychotherapy with hospitalized male inebriates. *Quarterly Journal of Studies on Alcohol, 18,* 263–277.

Erikson, E. H. (1963). *Childhood and society* (rev. ed.). New York: Norton.

Faber, E., & Keating-O'Connor, B. (1991). Planned family intervention: Johnson Institute method. *Journal of Chemical Dependency Treatment, 4,* 61–71.

Falkowski, W. (1996). Group therapy and the addictions. In G. Edwards & C. Dare (Eds.), *Psychotherapy, psychological treatments and the addictions* (pp. 206–219). Cambridge, UK: Cambridge University Press.

Fals-Stewart, W., Birchler, G. R., & O'Farrell, T. J. (1996). Behavioral couples therapy for male substance-abusing patients: Effects on relationship adjustment and drug-using behavior. *Journal of Consulting and Clinical Psychology, 64,* 959–972.

Fals-Stewart, W., O'Farrell, T. J., & Birchler, G. R. (1997). Behavioral couples therapy for male substance-abusing patients: A cost outcomes analysis. *Journal of Consulting and Clinical Psychology, 65,* 789–802.

Fals-Stewart, W., O'Farrell, T. J., Freitas, T., McFarlin, S. K., & Rutigliano, P. (2000). The timeline followback interview for substance abuse: Psychometric properties. *Journal of Consulting and Clinical Psychology, 68,* 134–144.

Famularo, R., Kinscherff, R., & Fenton, T. (1992). Parental substance abuse and the nature of child maltreatment. *Child Abuse and Neglect, 16,* 475–483.

Farkas, A. J., Pierce, J. P., Zhu, S. H., Rosbrook, B., Gilpin, E. A., Berry, C., & Kaplan, R. M. (1996). Addiction versus stages of change models in predicting smoking cessation. *Addiction, 91,* 1271–1280.

Fenichel, O. (1945). *The psychoanalytic theory of neurosis.* New York: Norton.

Finney, J. W., Moos, R. H., & Timko, C. (1999). The course of treated and untreated substance use disorders: Remission, resolution, relapse, and mortality. In B. S. McCrady & E. E. Epstein (Eds.), *Addiction: A comprehensive guidebook* (pp. 30–49). New York: Oxford University Press.

Flores, P. J. (1988). *Group psychotherapy with addicted populations.* New York: Haworth Press.

Frances, R. J., & Miller, S. I. (Eds.). (1991). *Clinical textbook of addictive disorders.* New York: Guilford Press.

Galanter, M., Castaneda, R., & Franco, H. (1991). Group therapy and self-help groups. In R. J. Frances & S. I. Miller (Eds.), *Clinical textbook of addictive disorders* (pp. 431–451). New York: Guilford Press.

Garrett, J., Landau, J., Shea, R., Stanton, M. D., Baciewicz, G., & Brinkman-Sull, D. (1998).

The ARISE intervention: Using family and network links to engage addicted persons in treatment. *Journal of Substance Abuse Treatment, 15*, 333–343.

Garrett, J., Landau-Stanton, J., Stanton, M. D., Stellato-Kabat, J., & Stellato-Kabat, D. (1997). ARISE: A method for engaging reluctant alcohol- and drug-dependent individuals in treatment. *Journal of Substance Abuse Treatment, 14*, 235–248.

Gentilello, L. M., Duggan, P., Drummond, D., Tonnesen, A., Degner, E. E., Fischer, R. P., & Reed, R. L. (1988). Major injury as a unique opportunity to initiate treatment in the alcoholic. *American Journal of Surgery, 156*, 558–561.

Gibbs, L. E. (1983). Validity and reliability of the Michigan Alcoholism Screening Test: A review. *Drug and Alcohol Dependence, 12*, 279–285.

Gillet, C., Paille, F., Wahl, D., Aubin, H. J., Pirolett, P., & Prime, T. (1991). Outcome of treatment in alcoholic women. *Drug and Alcohol Dependence, 29*, 189–194.

Gil-Rivas, V., Fiorentine, R., Anglin, M. D., & Taylor, E. (1997). Sexual and physical abuse: Do they compromise drug treatment outcomes? *Journal of Substance Abuse Treatment, 14*, 351–358.

Glynn, T. J., Boyd, G. M., & Gruman, J. C. (1990). Essential elements of self-help/minimal intervention strategies for smoking cessation. *Health Education Quarterly, 17*, 329–345.

Golden, S. J., Khantzian, E. J., & McAuliffe, W. E. (1994). Group therapy. In M. Galanter & H. D. Kleber (Eds.), *The American Psychiatric Press textbook of substance abuse treatment* (pp. 303–314). Washington, DC: American Psychiatric Press.

Golden, W. L. (1983). Resistance in cognitive-behavior therapy. *British Journal of Cognitive Psychotherapy, 1*, 33–42.

Goodwin, D. W., & Warnock, J. K. (1991). Alcoholism: A family disease. In R. J. Frances & S. I. Miller (Eds.), *Clinical textbook of addictive disorders* (pp. 485–500). New York: Guilford Press.

Gorski, T. T., & Miller, M. (1979). *Counseling for relapse prevention.* Hazel Creste, IL: Alcoholism Systems Associates.

Graham, J. R. (1999). *MMPI-2: Assessing personality and psychopathology* (3rd ed.). New York: Oxford University Press.

Graham, K., Annis, H. M., Brett, P. J., & Venesoen, P. (1996). A controlled field trial of group versus individual cognitive-behavioural training for relapse prevention. *Addiction, 91*, 1127–1140.

Greenson, R. R. (1967). *The technique and practice of psychoanalysis* (Vol. 1). New York: International Universities Press.

Grimley, D. M., Riley, G. E., Bellis, J. M., & Prochaska, J. O. (1993). Assessing the stages of change and decision-making for contraceptive use for the prevention of pregnancy, sexually transmitted diseases, and acquired immunodeficiency syndrome. *Health Education Quarterly, 20*, 455–470.

Gurman, A. S. (1984). Transference and resistance in marital therapy. *American Journal of Family Therapy, 12*, 70–73.

Hajek, P., Belcher, M., & Stapleton, J. (1985). Enhancing the impact of groups: An evaluation of two group formats for smokers. *British Journal of Clinical Psychology, 124*, 289–294.

Hartnoll, R. (1992). Research and the help-seeking process. *British Journal of Addiction, 87*, 429–437.

Harwood, H., Fountain, D., & Livermore, G. (1998). *The economic costs of alcohol and drug abuse in the United States—1992.* Rockville, MD: U.S. Department of Health and Human Services.

Hasin, D. S. (1991). Diagnostic interviews for assessment: Background, reliability, validity. *Alcohol Health and Research World, 15,* 293–302.

Hasin, D. S. (1994). Treatment/self-help for alcohol-related problems: Relationship to social pressure and alcohol dependence. *Journal of Studies on Alcohol, 55,* 660–666.

Hawkins, C. A. (1997). Disruption of family rituals as a mediator of the relationship between parental drinking and adult adjustment in offspring. *Addictive Behaviors, 22,* 219–231.

Heath, A. W., & Stanton, M. D. (1998). Family-based treatment: Stages and outcomes. *Clinical textbook of addictive disorders* (2nd ed., pp. 496–520). New York: Guilford Press.

Heather, N., Rollnick, S., & Bell, A. (1993). Predictive validity of the Readiness to Change Questionnaire. *Addiction, 88,* 1667–1677.

Heather, N., Stallard, A., & Tebbutt, J. (1991). Importance of substance cues in relapse among heroin users: Comparison of two methods of investigation. *Addictive Behaviors, 16,* 41–49.

Higgins, S. T. (1999). Potential contributions of the community reinforcement approach and contingency management to broadening the base of substance abuse treatment. In J. A. Tucker, D. M. Donovan, & G. A. Marlatt (Eds.), *Changing addictive behavior: Bridging clinical and public health strategies* (pp. 283–306). New York: Guilford Press.

Higgins, S. T., Tidey, J. W., & Stitzer, M. L. (1998). Community reinforcement and contingency management interventions. In A. W. Graham, T. K. Schultz, & B. B. Wilford (Eds.), *Principles of addiction medicine* (pp. 675–690). Chevy Chase, MD: American Society of Addiction Medicine.

Hingson, R., Mangione, T., Meyers, A., & Scotch, N. (1982). Seeking help for drinking problems. *Journal of Studies on Alcohol, 43,* 273–288.

Hinkin, C. H., & Kahn, M. (1995). Psychological symptomatology in spouses and adult children of alcoholics: An examination of the hypothesized personality characteristics of codependency. *International Journal of the Addictions, 30,* 843–861.

Hodgins, D. C., el-Guebaly, N., & Addington, J. (1997). Treatment of substance abusers: Single or mixed gender programs? *Addiction, 92,* 805–812.

Hoffman, J. A., Caudill, B. D., Koman, J. J., Luckey, J. W., Flynn, P. M., & Hubbard, R. L. (1994). Comparative cocaine abuse treatment strategies: Enhancing client retention and treatment exposure. *Journal of Addictive Diseases, 13,* 115–128.

Holder, H. D. (1998). The cost offsets of alcoholism treatment. In M. Galanter (Ed.), *Recent developments in alcoholism* (Vol. 14, pp. 361–374). New York: Plenum Press.

Holder, H. D., Lennox, R. D., & Blose, J. O. (1992). The economic benefits of alcoholism treatment: A summary of twenty years of research. *Journal of Employee Assistance Research, 1,* 63–82.

Horn, D. A. (1976). A model for the study of personal choice health behavior. *International Journal of Health Education, 19,* 89–98.

Horn, J. L., Wanberg, K. W., & Foster, F. M. (1987). *Guide to the Alcohol Use Inventory (AUI).* Minneapolis, MN: National Computer Systems.

Hubbard, R. L., Marsden, M. E., Rachal, J. V., Harwood, H. J., Cavanaugh, E. R., &

Ginzburg, H. M. (1989). *Drug abuse treatment: A national study of effectiveness.* Chapel Hill: University of North Carolina Press.

Humphreys, K., & Moos, R. H. (1996). Reduced substance-abuse-related health care costs among voluntary participants in Alcoholics Anonymous. *Psychiatric Services, 47,* 709–713.

Hunt, G. M., & Azrin, N. H. (1973). A community-reinforcement approach to alcoholism. *Behaviour Research and Therapy, 11,* 91–104.

Hunt, W. A., Barnett, L. W., & Branch, L. G. (1971). Relapse rates in addiction programs. *Journal of Clinical Psychology, 27,* 455–456.

Iguchi, M. Y., Belding, M. A., Morral, A. R., Lamb, R. J., & Husband, S. D. (1997). Reinforcing operants other than abstinence in drug abuse treatment: An effective alternative for reducing drug use. *Journal of Consulting and Clinical Psychology, 65,* 421–428.

Institute of Medicine. (1990). *Broadening the base of treatment for alcohol problems.* Washington, DC: National Academy Press.

Ireland, T., & Widom, C. S. (1994). Childhood victimization and risk for alcohol and drug arrests. *International Journal of the Addictions, 29,* 235–274.

Isenhart, C. E. (1991). Factor structure of the Inventory of Drinking Situations. *Journal of Substance Abuse, 3,* 59–71.

Isenhart, C. E. (1993). Psychometric evaluation of a short form of the Inventory of Drinking Situations. *Journal of Studies on Alcohol, 54,* 345–349.

Isenhart, C. (1994). Motivational subtypes in an inpatient sample of substance abusers. *Addictive Behaviors, 19,* 463–475.

Ito, J. R., Donovan, D. M., & Hall, J. J. (1988). Relapse prevention in alcohol after-care: Effects on drinking outcome, change process, and after-care attendance. *British Journal of Addiction, 83,* 171–181.

Jacobson, G. R. (1989). A comprehensive approach to pretreatment evaluation: I. Detection, assessment, and diagnosis of alcoholism. In R. K. Hester & W. R. Miller (Eds.), *Handbook of alcoholism treatment approaches* (pp. 17–53). New York: Pergamon Press.

Jahn, D. L., & Lichstein, K. L. (1980). The resistive client: A neglected phenomenon in behavior therapy. *Behavior Modification, 4,* 303–320.

Janis, I. L., & Mann, L. (1977). *Decision-making: A psychological analysis of conflict, choice, and commitment.* New York: Free Press.

Johnson, V. E. (1986). *Intervention: How to help someone who doesn't want help.* Minneapolis, MN: Johnson Institute Books.

Joint Commission on Accreditation of Healthcare Organizations. (1994). *Accreditation manual for mental health, chemical dependency, and mental retardation/developmental disabilities services.* Oakbrook Terrace, IL: Author.

Joint Commission on Accreditation of Healthcare Organizations. (1996). *1997–98 comprehensive accreditation manual for behavioral health care.* Oakbrook Terrace, IL: Author.

Jordan, C. M., & Oei, T. P. S. (1989). Help-seeking behaviour in problem drinkers: A review. *British Journal of Addiction, 84,* 979–988.

Joseph, J., Breslin, C., & Skinner, H. (1999). Critical perspectives on the transtheoretical model and stages of change. In J. A. Tucker, D. M. Donovan, & G. A. Marlatt (Eds.), *Changing addictive behavior: Bridging clinical and public health strategies* (pp. 160–190). New York: Guilford Press.

Kadden, R., Carroll, K., Donovan, D., Cooney, N., Monti, P., Abrams, D., Litt, M., & Hester, R. (1992). *Cognitive-behavioral coping skills therapy manual: A clinical research guide for therapists treating individuals with alcohol abuse and dependence* (National Institute on Alcohol Abuse and Alcoholism, Project MATCH Monograph Series, Vol. 3). Rockville, MD: National Institute on Alcohol Abuse and Alcoholism.

Kanfer, F. H. (1986). Implications of a self-regulation model of therapy for treatment of addictive behaviors. In W. R. Miller & N. Heather (Eds.), *Treating addictive behaviors: Processes of change*. New York: Plenum Press.

Kaskutas, L. A. (1996a). Road less traveled: Choosing the "Women for Sobriety" program. *Journal of Drug Issues, 26,* 77–94.

Kaskutas, L. A. (1996b). Pathways to self-help among Women for Sobriety. *American Journal of Drug and Alcohol Abuse, 22,* 259–280.

Kauffman, E., Dore, M. M., & Nelson-Zlupko, L. (1995). The role of women's therapy groups in the treatment of chemical dependence. *American Journal of Orthopsychiatry, 65,* 355–363.

Kaufman, E. (1994). *Psychotherapy of addicted persons.* New York: Guilford Press.

Kaufman, E., & Reoux, J. (1988). Guidelines for the successful psychotherapy of substance abusers. *American Journal of Drug and Alcohol Abuse, 14,* 199–209.

Kelleher, K., Chaffin, M., Hollenberg, J., & Fischer, E. (1994). Alcohol and drug disorders among physically abusive and neglectful parents in a community-based sample. *American Journal of Public Health, 84,* 1586–1590.

Kirby, K. C., Marlowe, D. B., Festinger, D. S., Garvey, K. A., & LaMonaca, V. (1999). Community reinforcement training for family and significant others of drug abusers: A unilateral intervention to increase treatment entry of drug abusers. *Drug and Alcohol Dependence, 56,* 85–96.

Klingemann, H. (1991). The motivation for change from problem alcohol and heroin use. *British Journal of Addiction, 86,* 727–744.

Kofoed, L. (1993). Outpatient vs. inpatient treatment for the chronically mentally ill with substance use disorders. *Journal of Addictive Diseases, 12,* 123–127.

Kofoed, L. (1997). Engagement and persuasion. In N. S. Miller (Ed.), *The principles and practice of addictions in psychiatry* (pp. 214–220). Philadelphia: Saunders.

Krampen, G. (1989). Motivation in the treatment of alcoholism. *Addictive Behaviors, 14,* 197–200.

Kurtz, P. D., Gaudin, J. M., Howing, P. T., & Wodarski, J. S. (1993). The consequences of physical abuse and neglect on the school age child: Mediating factors. *Children and Youth Services Review, 15,* 85–104.

Larson, C. C., & Talley, L. K. (1977). Family resistance to therapy: A model for services and therapists' roles. *Child Welfare, 56,* 121–126.

Lazarus, A. A., & Fay, A. (1982). Resistance or rationalization?: A cognitive-behavioral perspective. In P. L. Wachtel (Ed.), *Resistance: Psychodynamic and behavioral approaches* (pp. 115–132). New York: Plenum Press.

Lehman, A. F., Myers, C. P., Corty, E., & Thompson, J. W. (1994). Prevalence and patterns of "dual diagnosis" among psychiatric inpatients. *Comprehensive Psychiatry, 35,* 106–112.

Lehman, A. F., Myers, C. P., Dixon, L. B., & Johnson, J. L. (1994). Defining subgroups of dual diagnosis patients for service planning. *Hospital and Community Psychiatry, 45,* 556–561.

Lehman, A. F., Myers, C. P., Thompson, J. W., & Corty, E. (1993). Implications of mental and substance use disorders: A comparison of single and dual diagnosis patients. *Journal of Nervous and Mental Disease, 181,* 365–370.

Leigh, G., & Skinner, H. A. (1988). Physiological assessment. In D. M. Donovan & G. A. Marlatt (Eds.), *Assessment of addictive behaviors* (pp. 112–136). New York: Guilford Press.

Lemmens, P., Tan, E. S., & Knibbe, R. A. (1992). Measuring quantity and frequency of drinking in a general population survey: A comparison of five indices. *Journal of Studies on Alcohol, 53,* 476–486.

Lennox, R. D., Scott-Lennox, J. A., & Bohlig, E. M. (1993). The cost of depression-complicated alcoholism: Health-care utilization and treatment effectiveness. *Journal of Mental Health Administration, 20,* 138–152.

Levy, M. (1997). Group therapy in addictive and psychiatric disorders. In N. S. Miller (Ed.), *The principles and practice of addictions in psychiatry* (pp. 384–391). Philadelphia: Saunders.

Lewis, J. A., Dana, R. Q., & Blevins, G. A. (1988). *Substance abuse counseling: An individualized approach.* Pacific Grove, CA: Brooks/Cole.

Lichtenstein, E. (1971). Modification of smoking behavior: Good designs—ineffective treatment. *Journal of Consulting and Clinical Psychology, 36,* 163–166.

Liepman, M. R. (1993). Using family influence to motivate alcoholics to enter treatment: The Johnson Institute Intervention approach. In T. J. O'Farrell (Ed.), *Treating alcohol problems: Marital and family interventions* (pp. 54–77). New York: Guilford Press.

Litman, G. K. (1986). Alcoholism survival: The prevention of relapse. In W. R. Miller & N. Heather (Eds.), *Treating addictive behaviors* (pp. 391–405). New York: Plenum Press.

Litman, G. K., Eiser, J. R., Rawson, N. S. B., & Oppenheim, A. N. (1979). Towards a typology of relapse: Differences in relapse and coping behaviours between alcoholic relapsers and survivors. *Behaviour Research and Therapy, 17,* 89–94.

Loneck, B., Garrett, J. A., & Banks, S. M. (1996). A comparison of the Johnson intervention with four other methods of referral to outpatient treatment. *American Journal of Drug and Alcohol Abuse, 22,* 233–246.

Loneck, B., Garrett, J., & Banks, S. M. (1997). Engaging and retaining women in outpatient alcohol and other drug treatment: The effect of referral intensity. *Health and Social Work, 22,* 38–46.

Longabaugh, R., Wirtz, P. W., Beattie, M. C., Noel, N., & Stout, R. (1995). Matching treatment focus to patient social investment and support: 18 month follow-up results. *Journal of Consulting and Clinical Psychology, 63,* 296–307.

Lotti, G. (1987). The resistance to change of cognitive structures: A counterproposal to psychoanalytic metapsychology. *Journal of Cognitive Psychotherapy, 1,* 87–104.

Lovejoy, M., Rosenblum, A., Magura, S., Foote, J., Handelsman, L., & Stimmel, B. (1995). Patients' perspective on the process of change in substance abuse treatment. *Journal of Substance Abuse Treatment, 12,* 269–282.

Lovett, L., & Lovett, J. (1991). Group therapeutic factors on an alcohol in-patient unit. *British Journal of Psychiatry, 159,* 365–370.

Luborsky, L., Singer, B., & Luborsky, L. (1975). Comparative studies of psychotherapy: Is it true that "Everyone has won and all must get prizes"? *Archives of General Psychiatry, 32,* 995–1008.

Ludwig, A. M., & Wikler, A. (1974). "Craving" and relapse to drink. *Quarterly Journal of Studies on Alcohol, 35,* 108–130.

Lutz, M. E. (1991). Sobering decisions: Are there gender differences? *Alcoholism Treatment Quarterly, 8,* 51–64.

MacAndrew, C. (1965). The differentiation of male alcoholic outpatients from non-alcoholic psychiatric outpatients by means of the MMPI. *Quarterly Journal of Studies on Alcohol, 26,* 238–246.

Magura, S., Casriel, C., Goldsmith, D. S., & Lipton, D. S. (1987). Contracting with clients in methadone treatment. *Social Casework, 68,* 485–493.

Magura, S., Casriel, C., Goldsmith, D. S., Strug, D. L., & Lipton, D. S. (1988). Contingency contracting with polydrug-abusing methadone patients. *Addictive Behaviors, 13,* 113–118.

Maisto, S. A., & Connors, G. J. (1990). Clinical diagnostic techniques and assessment tools in alcohol research. *Alcohol Health and Research World, 14,* 232–238.

Maisto, S. A., McKay, J. R., & Connors, G. J. (1990). Self-report issues in substance abuse: State of the art and future directions. *Behavioral Assessment, 12,* 117–134.

Maisto, S. A., O'Farrell, T. J., Worthen, M., & Walitzer, K. S. (1993). Alcohol abuse and dependence. In A. S. Bellack & M. Hersen (Eds.), *Handbook of behavior therapy in the psychiatric setting* (pp. 293–319). New York: Plenum Press.

Mallams, J. H., Godley, M. D., Hall, G. M., & Meyers, R. J. (1982). A social-systems approach to resocializing alcoholics in the community. *Journal of Studies on Alcohol, 43,* 1115–1123.

Marcus, B. H., Rossi, J. S., Selby, V. C., Niaura, R. S., & Abrams, D. B. (1992). The stages and processes of exercise adoption and maintenance in a worksite sample. *Health Psychology, 11,* 386–395.

Mark, F. O. (1988). Does coercion work? The role of referral source in motivating alcoholics in treatment. *Alcoholism Treatment Quarterly, 5,* 5–22.

Marlatt, G. A. (1985a). Lifestyle modification. In G. A. Marlatt & J. R. Gordon (Eds.), *Relapse prevention* (pp. 280–348). New York: Guilford Press.

Marlatt, G. A. (1985b). Relapse prevention: Theoretical rationale and overview of the model. In G. A. Marlatt & J. R. Gordon (Eds.), *Relapse prevention* (pp. 3–70). New York: Guilford Press.

Marlatt, G. A. (1996). Taxonomy of high-risk situations for alcohol relapse: Evolution and development of a cognitive-behavioral model. *Addiction, 91*(Suppl.), 37–49.

Marlatt, G. A., & Gordon, J. R. (1980). Determinants of relapse: Implications for the maintenance of behavior change. In P. O. Davidson & S. M. Davidson (Eds.), *Behavioral medicine: Changing health lifestyles* (pp. 410–452). New York: Brunner/Mazel.

Marlatt, G. A., & Gordon, J. R. (Eds.). (1985). *Relapse prevention.* New York: Guilford Press.

Marlatt, G. A., Tucker, J. A., Donovan, D. M., & Vuchinich, R. E. (1997). Help-seeking by substance abusers: The role of harm reduction and behavioral-economic approaches to facilitate treatment entry and retention. In L. S. Onken, J. D. Blaine, & J. J. Boren (Eds.), *Beyond the therapeutic alliance: Keeping the drug-dependent individual in treatment* (pp. 44–84). Rockville, MD: National Institute on Drug Abuse.

Martin, G. W., & Wilkinson, D. A. (1989). Methodological issues in the evaluation of treatment of drug dependence. *Behaviour Research and Therapy, 11,* 133–150.

Martin, K., Giannandrea, P., Rogers, B., & Johnson, J. (1996). Group intervention with pre-recovery patients. *Journal of Substance Abuse Treatment, 13*, 33–41.

Matano, R. A., & Yalom, I. D. (1991). Approaches to chemical dependency: Chemical dependency and interactive group therapy—a synthesis. *International Journal of Group Psychotherapy, 41*, 269–293.

Mayer, J. E., & Koeningsmark, C. S. (1991). Self-efficacy, relapse and the possibility of posttreatment denial as a stage in alcoholism. *Alcoholism Treatment Quarterly, 8*, 1–16.

Mayfield, D., McLeod, G., & Hall, P. (1974). The CAGE questionnaire: Validation of a new alcoholism instrument. *American Journal of Psychiatry, 131*, 1121–1123.

McConnaughy, E. A., DiClemente, C. C., Prochaska, J. O., & Velicer, W. F. (1989). Stages of change in psychotherapy: A follow-up report. *Psychotherapy, 26*, 494–503.

McConnaughy, E. A., Prochaska, J. O., & Velicer, W. F. (1983). Stages of change in psychotherapy: Measurement and sample profiles. *Psychotherapy: Theory, Research and Practice, 20*, 368–375.

McCrady, B. S. (1989). Extending relapse prevention models to couples. *Addictive Behaviors, 14*, 69–74.

McCrady, B. S. (1991). Promising but underutilized treatment approaches. *Alcohol Health and Research World, 15*, 215–218.

McCrady, B. S. (1993). Relapse prevention: A couples-therapy perspective. In T. J. O'Farrell (Ed.), *Treating alcohol problems: Marital and family interventions* (pp. 327–350). New York: Guilford Press.

McCrady, B. S., Noel, N. E., Abrams, D. B., Stout, R. L., Neben, H. F., & Hay, W. M. (1986). Comparative effectiveness of three types of spouse involvement in outpatient behavioral alcoholism treatment. *Journal of Studies on Alcohol, 47*, 459–467.

McCrady, B. S., & Raytek, H. (1993). Women and substance abuse: Treatment modalities and outcomes. In E. S. L. Gomberg & T. D. Nirenberg (Eds.), *Women and substance abuse* (pp. 314–338). Norwood, NJ: Ablex Publishing Corp.

McCrady, B. S., Stout, R., Noel, N., Abrams, D., & Fisher-Nelson, H. (1991). Effectiveness of three types of spouse-involved behavioral alcoholism treatment. *British Journal of Addiction, 86*, 1415–1424.

McDuff, D., & Muneses, T. I. (1998). Mental health strategy: Addiction interventions for the dually diagnosed. In R. K. White & D. G. Wright (Eds.), *Addiction intervention: Strategies to motivate treatment-seeking behavior* (pp. 37–53). New York: Haworth Press.

McGaha, J. E., & Leoni, E. L. (1995). Family violence, abuse, and related family issues of incarcerated delinquents with alcoholic parents compared to those with non-alcoholic parents. *Adolescence, 30*, 473–482.

McGue, M. (1997). A behavioral-genetic perspective on children of alcoholics. *Alcohol Health and Research World, 21*, 210–217.

McKay, J. R., Maisto, S. A., & O'Farrell, T. J., (1996). Alcoholics' perceptions of factors in the onset and termination of relapses and the maintenance of abstinence: Results from a 30-month follow-up, *Psychology of Addictive Behaviors, 10*, 167–180.

McKay, J. R., Rutherford, M. J., Cacciola, J. S., Kabasakalian-McKay, R., & Alterman, A. I. (1996). Gender differences in the relapse experiences of cocaine patients. *Journal of Nervous and Mental Disease, 184*, 616–622.

McLellan, A. T., Alterman, A. I., Metzger, D. S., Grissom, G. R., Woody, G. E., Luborsky, L., & O'Brien, C. P. (1994) Similarity of outcome predictors across opiate, cocaine and alcohol treatments: Role of treatment services. *Journal of Consulting and Clinical Psychology, 62,* 1141–1158.

McLellan, A., Arndt, I., Metzger, D., Woody, G., & O'Brien, C. (1993). The effects of psychosocial services in substance abuse treatment. *Journal of the American Medical Association, 269,* 1953–1959.

McLellan, A. T., Kushner, H., Metzger, D., Peters, R., Smith, I., Grissom, G., Pettinati, H., & Argeriou, M. (1992). The fifth edition of the Addiction Severity Index. *Journal of Substance Abuse Treatment, 9,* 199–213.

McLellan, A. T., Luborsky, L., Woody, G. E., & O'Brien, C. P. (1980). An improved diagnostic evaluation instrument for substance abuse patients: The Addiction Severity Index. *Journal of Nervous and Mental Disease, 168,* 26–33.

Meichenbaum, D. H. (1995). Cognitive-behavioral therapy in historical perspective. In B. Bongar & L. E. Beutler (Eds.), *Comprehensive textbook of psychotherapy* (pp. 140–158). New York: Oxford University Press.

Merikangas, K. R. (1990). Genetic epidemiology of alcoholism. *Psychological Medicine, 20,* 1–22.

Metzger, L. (1988). *From denial to recovery.* San Francisco: Jossey-Bass.

Meyers, R. J., Smith, J. E., & Miller, E. J. (1998). Working through the concerned significant other. In W. R. Miller & N. Heather (Eds.), *Treating addictive behaviors* (2nd ed., pp. 149–161). New York: Plenum Press.

Milby, J. B., Schumacher, J. E., Raczynski, J. M., Caldwell, E., Engle, M., Michael, M., & Carr, J. (1996). Sufficient conditions for effective treatment of substance abusing homeless persons. *Drug and Alcohol Dependence, 43,* 39–47.

Milgram, D., & Rubin, J. S. (1992). Resisting resistance: Involuntary substance abuse group therapy. *Social Work with Groups, 15,* 95–110.

Miller, K. J., McCrady, B. S., Abrams, D. B., & Labouvie, E. W. (1994). Taking an individualized approach to the assessment of self-efficacy and the prediction of alcoholic relapse. *Journal of Psychopathology and Behavioral Assessment, 16,* 111–120.

Miller, N. S. (1995). Group therapy. In N. S. Miller (Ed.), *Addiction psychiatry: Current diagnoses and treatment* (pp. 256–270). New York: Wiley.

Miller, P. J., Ross, S. M., Emmerson, R. Y., & Todt, E. H. (1989). Self-efficacy in alcoholics: Clinical validation of the Situational Confidence Questionnaire. *Addictive Behaviors, 14,* 217–224.

Miller, P. M., & Mastria, M. A. (1977). *Alternatives to alcohol abuse: A social learning model.* Champaign, IL: Research Press.

Miller, W. R. (1985). Motivation for treatment: A review with special emphasis on alcoholism. *Psychological Bulletin, 98,* 84–107.

Miller, W. R. (1992). The effectiveness of treatment for substance abuse: Reasons for optimism. *Journal of Substance Abuse Treatment, 9,* 93–102.

Miller, W. R. (1995). Increasing motivation for change. In R. K. Hester & W. R. Miller (Eds.), *Handbook of alcoholism treatment approaches: Effective alternatives* (2nd ed., pp. 89–104). Boston: Allyn & Bacon.

Miller, W. R. (1996). *Manual for Form 90: A structured assessment interview for drinking and related behaviors* (National Institute on Alcohol Abuse and Alcoholism, Project MATCH Monograph Series, Vol. 5). Rockville, MD: National Institute on Alcohol Abuse and Alcoholism.

Miller, W. R. (Consensus Panel Chair). (1999). *Enhancing motivation for change in substance abuse treatment* (DHHS Publication No. (SMA) 99–3354; CSAT Treatment Improvement Protocol No. 35). Washington, DC: U. S. Government Printing Office.

Miller, W. R., Benefield, R. G., & Tonigan, J. S. (1993). Enhancing motivation for change in problem drinking: A controlled comparison of two therapist styles. *Journal of Consulting and Clinical Psychology, 61,* 455–461.

Miller, W. R., Brown, J. M., Simpson, T. L., Handmaker, N. S., Bien, T. H., Luckie, L. F., Montgomery, H. A., Hester, R. K., & Tonigan, J. S. (1995). What works? A methodological analysis of the alcohol treatment outcome literature. In R. K. Hester & W. R. Miller (Eds.), *Handbook of alcoholism treatment approaches: Effective alternatives* (2nd ed., pp. 12–44). Boston: Allyn & Bacon.

Miller, W. R., & DelBoca, F. K. (1994). Measurement of drinking behavior using the Form 90 family of instruments. *Journal of Studies on Alcohol,* Suppl. 12, 112–118.

Miller, W. R., & Hester, R. K. (1980). Treating the problem drinker: Modern approaches. In W. R. Miller (Ed.), *The addictive behaviors: Treatment of alcoholism, drug abuse, smoking, and obesity* (pp. 11–141). New York: Pergamon Press.

Miller, W. R., & Hester, R. K. (1986). The effectiveness of alcoholism treatment: What research reveals. In W. R. Miller & N. Heather (Eds.), *Treating addictive behaviors: Processes of change* (pp. 121–174). New York: Plenum Press.

Miller, W. R., Leckman, A. L., Delaney, H. D., & Tinkcom, M. (1992). Long-term follow-up of behavioral self-control training. *Journal of Studies on Alcohol, 53,* 249–261.

Miller, W. R., & Marlatt, G. A. (1984). *Manual for the Comprehensive Drinker Profile.* Odessa, FL: Psychological Assessment Resources.

Miller, W. R., Meyers, R. J., & Tonigan, J. S. (1999). Engaging the unmotivated in treatment for alcohol problems: A comparison of three strategies for intervention through family members. *Journal of Consulting and Clinical Psychology, 67,* 688–697.

Miller, W. R., & Rollnick, S. (1991). *Motivational interviewing: Preparing people to change addictive behavior.* New York: Guilford Press.

Miller, W. R., & Sanchez, V. C. (1994). Motivating young adults for treatment and lifestyle change. In G. Howard (Ed.), *Issues in alcohol use and misuse by young adults* (pp. 55–82). Notre Dame, IN: University of Notre Dame Press.

Miller, W. R., & Tonigan, J. S. (1996). Assessing drinkers' motivations for change: The Stages of Change Readiness and Eagerness Scale (SOCRATES). *Psychology of Addictive Behaviors, 10,* 81–89.

Miller, W. R., Westerberg, V. S., Harris, R. J., & Tonigan, J. S. (1996). What predicts relapse? Prospective testing of antecedent models. *Addiction, 91*(Suppl.), 155–171.

Miller, W. R., Zweben, A., DiClemente, C. C., & Rychtarik, R. G. (1992). *Motivational enhancement therapy manual: A clinical research guide for therapists treating individuals with alcohol abuse and dependence* (National Institute on Alcohol Abuse and Alcoholism, Project MATCH Monograph Series, Vol. 2). Rockville, MD: National Institute on Alcohol Abuse and Alcoholism.

Monti, P. M., Abrams, D. B., Kadden, R. M., & Cooney, N. L. (1989). *Treating alcohol dependence.* New York: Guilford Press.

Moos, R. H., Finney, J. W., & Cronkite, R. C. (1990). *Alcoholism treatment: Context, process, and outcome.* New York: Oxford University Press.

Morse, R. M., & Flavin, D. K. (1992). The definition of alcoholism. *Journal of the American Medical Association, 268,* 1012–1014.

Muetzell, S. (1995). Are boys more vulnerable than girls in alcoholic families? *Early Child Development and Care, 105,* 43–58.

Muhleman, D. (1987). 12-step study groups in drug abuse treatment programs. *Journal of Psychoactive Drugs, 19,* 291–298.

Murphy, C. M., & O'Farrell, T. J. (1996). Marital violence among alcoholics. *Current Directions in Psychological Science, 5,* 183–186.

Murphy, C. M., & O'Farrell, T. J. (1997). Couple communication patterns of maritally aggressive and nonaggressive male alcoholics. *Journal of Studies on Alcohol, 58,* 83–90.

Nelson-Zlupko, L., Dore, M. M., Kauffman, E., & Kaltenbach, K. (1996). Women in recovery: Their perceptions of treatment effectiveness. *Journal of Substance Abuse Treatment, 13,* 51–59.

Niles, B. L., & McCrady, B. S. (1991). Detection of alcohol problems in a hospital setting. *Addictive Behaviors, 16,* 223–233.

Norcross, J. C., & Goldfried, M. R. (Eds.). (1992). *Handbook of psychotherapy integration.* New York: Basic Books.

Nordstrom, G., & Berglund, M. (1987). A prospective study of successful long-term adjustment in alcohol dependence: Social drinking versus abstinence. *Journal of Studies on Alcohol, 48,* 95–103.

Nowinski, J. (1999). Self-help groups for addictions. In B. S. McCrady & E. E. Epstein (Eds.), *Addiction: A comprehensive guidebook* (pp. 328–346). New York: Oxford University Press.

Obert, J. L., Rawson, R. A., & Miotto, K. (1997). Substance abuse treatment for "hazardous users": An early intervention. *Journal of Psychoactive Drugs, 29,* 291–298.

O'Brien, C. P. (1996). Recent developments in the pharmacotherapy of substance abuse. *Journal of Consulting and Clinical Psychology, 64,* 677–686.

O'Farrell, T. J. (1989). Marital and family therapy in alcoholism treatment. *Journal of Substance Abuse Treatment, 6,* 23–29.

O'Farrell, T. J. (1993a). Couples relapse prevention sessions after a behavioral marital therapy couples group program. In T. J. O'Farrell (Ed.), *Treating alcohol problems: Marital and family interventions* (pp. 305–326). New York: Guilford Press.

O'Farrell, T. J. (Ed.). (1993b). *Treating alcohol problems: Marital and family interventions.* New York: Guilford Press.

O'Farrell, T. J., & Bayog, R. D. (1986). Antabuse contracts for married alcoholics and their spouses: A method to maintain Antabuse ingestion and decrease conflict about drinking. *Journal of Substance Abuse Treatment, 3,* 1–8.

O'Farrell, T. J., Choquette, K. A., & Cutter, H. S. (1998). Couples relapse prevention sessions after behavioral marital therapy for male alcoholics: Outcomes during the three years after starting treatment. *Journal of Studies on Alcohol, 59,* 357–370.

O'Farrell, T. J., Choquette, K. A., Cutter, H. S., Brown, E. D., & McCourt, W. F. (1993). Behavioral marital therapy with and without additional couples relapse prevention sessions for alcoholics and their wives. *Journal of Studies on Alcohol, 54,* 652–666.

O'Farrell, T. J., & Cowles, K. S. (1989). Marital and family therapy. In R. K. Hester & W. R. Miller (Eds.), *Handbook of alcoholism treatment approaches: Effective alternatives* (pp. 183–205). Elmsford, NY: Pergamon Press.

O'Farrell, T. J., Cutter, H. S., Choquette, K. A., Floyd, F. J., & Bayog, R. D. (1992). Behavioral marital therapy for male alcoholics: Marital and drinking adjustment during the two years after treatment. *Behavior Therapy, 23,* 529–549.

O'Farrell, T. J., & Feehan, M. (1999). Alcoholism treatment and the family: Do family and individual treatments for alcoholic adults have preventive effects for children? *Journal of Studies on Alcohol, 13,* 125–129.

Olsen, L. J. (1995). Services for substance abuse-affected families: The Project Connect experience. *Child and Adolescent Social Work Journal, 12,* 183–196.

O'Malley, S. S. (June 2000). COMBINE: Overview of the study design. In S. S. O'Malley & M. Mattson (Chairs), *Design and rationale for COMBINE: A multi-site study on combining medications and behavioral interventions for alcohol dependence.* Symposium presented at the annual meeting of the Research Society on Alcoholism, Denver, CO.

Oppenheimer, E. (1991). Alcohol and drug misuse among women: An overview. *British Journal of Psychiatry, 158*(Suppl. 10), 36–44.

Orford, J., & Edwards, G. (1977). *Alcoholism: A comparison of treatment and advice, with a study of influence of marriage* (Maudsley Monographs No. 26). New York: Oxford University Press.

Orford, J., & Keddie, A. (1986). Abstinence or controlled drinking in clinical practice: Indications at initial assessment. *Addictive Behaviors, 11,* 71–86.

Osher, F. C., & Kofoed, L. L. (1989). Treatment of patients with psychiatric and psychoactive substance abuse disorders. *Hospital and Community Psychiatry, 40,* 1025–1030.

Ossip-Klein, D. J., & Rychtarik, R. G. (1993). Behavioral contracts between alcoholics and family members: Improving aftercare participation and maintaining sobriety after inpatient alcoholism treatment. In T. J. O'Farrell (Eds.), *Treating alcohol problems: Marital and family interventions* (pp. 281–304). New York: Guilford Press.

Ossip-Klein, D. J., Vanlandingham, W., Prue, D. M., & Rychtarik, R. G. (1984). Increasing attendance at alcohol aftercare using calendar prompts and home based contracting. *Addictive Behaviors, 9,* 85–89.

Paolino, T. J., & McCrady, B. S. (1977). *The alcoholic marriage: Alternative perspectives.* New York: Grune & Stratton.

Perz, C. A., DiClemente, C. C., & Carbonari, J. P. (1996). Doing the right thing at the right time? Interaction of stages and processes of change in successful smoking cessation. *Health Psychology, 15,* 462–468.

Peters, R. H., & Schonfeld, L. (1993). Determinants of recent substance abuse among jail inmates referred for treatment. *Journal of Drug Issues, 23,* 101–117.

Peterson, K. A., Swindle, R. W., Phibbs, C. S., Recine, B., & Moos, R. H. (1994). Determinants of readmission following inpatient substance abuse treatment: A national study of VA programs. *Medical Care, 32,* 535–550.

Piazza, N. J., Vrbka, J. L., & Yeager, R. D. (1989). Telescoping of alcoholism in women alcoholics. *International Journal of the Addictions, 24,* 19–28.

Pierce, J. P., Farkas, A., Zhu, S-H., Berry, C., & Kaplan, R. M. (1996) Should the stage of change model be challenged? *Addiction, 91,* 1290–1293.

Pokorny, A. D., Miller, B. A., & Kaplan, H. B. (1972). The brief MAST: A shortened version of the Michigan Alcoholism Screening Test. *American Journal of Psychiatry, 129,* 342–345.

Polich, J. M., Armor, D. J., & Braiker, H. B. (1981). *The course of alcoholism: Four years after treatment*. New York: Wiley.

Pollock, V. E., Schneider, L. S., Gabrielli, W. F., & Goodwin, D. W. (1987). Sex of parent and offspring in the transmission of alcoholism: A meta-analysis. *Journal of Nervous and Mental Disease, 175*, 668–673.

Price, R. H., Burke, A. C., D'Aunno, T. A., Klingel, D. M., McCaughrin, W. C., Rafferty, J. A., & Vaughn, T. E. (1991). Outpatient drug abuse treatment services, 1988: Results of a national survey. In R. W. Pickens, C. G. Leukefeld, & C. R. Schuster (Eds.), *Improving drug abuse treatment* (pp. 63–92). Rockville, MD: National Institute on Drug Abuse.

Price, R. K., Cottler, L. B., & Robins, L. N. (1991). Patterns of drug abuse treatment utilization in a general population. In L. Harris (Ed.), *Problems of drug dependence, 1990* (pp. 466–467). Washington, DC: U.S. Government Printing Office.

Prochaska, J. O. (1979). *Systems of psychotherapy: A transtheoretical analysis*. Homewood, IL: Dorsey Press.

Prochaska, J. O. (1984). *Systems of psychotherapy: A transtheoretical analysis* (2nd ed.). Homewood, IL: Dorsey Press.

Prochaska, J. O. (1994). Strong and weak principles for progressing from precontemplation to action on the basis of twelve problem behaviors. *Health Psychology, 13*, 47–51.

Prochaska, J. O., & DiClemente, C. C. (1982). Transtheoretical therapy: Toward a more integrative model of change. *Psychotherapy: Theory, Research and Practice, 19*, 276–288.

Prochaska, J. O., & DiClemente, C. C. (1983). Stages and processes of self-change of smoking: Toward an integrative model of change. *Journal of Consulting and Clinical Psychology, 51*, 390–395.

Prochaska, J. O., & DiClemente, C. C. (1984). *The transtheoretical approach: Crossing the traditional boundaries of therapy*. Malabar, FL: Krieger.

Prochaska, J. O., & DiClemente, C. C. (1986). Toward a comprehensive model of change. In W. R. Miller & N. Heather (Eds.), *Treating addictive behaviors: Processes of change* (pp. 3–27). New York: Plenum Press.

Prochaska, J. O., & DiClemente, C. C. (1992). Stages of change in the modification of problem behaviors. In M. Hersen, R. M. Eisler, & P. M. Miller (Eds.), *Progress in behavior modification* (Vol. 28, pp. 183–218). Sycamore, IL: Sycamore Publishing Co.

Prochaska, J. O., & DiClemente, C. C. (1998). Comments, criteria and creating better models. In W. R. Miller & N. Heather (Eds.), *Treating addictive behaviors* (2nd ed., pp. 39–45). New York: Plenum.

Prochaska, J. O., DiClemente, C. C., & Norcross, J. C. (1992). In search of how people change: Applications to addictive behaviors. *American Psychologist, 47*, 1102–1114.

Prochaska, J. O., DiClemente, C. C., Velicer, W. F., & Rossi, J. S. (1993). Standardized, individualized, interactive and personalized self-help programs for smoking cessation. *Health Psychology, 12*, 399–405.

Prochaska, J. O., Johnson, S., & Lee, P. (1998). The transtheoretical model of behavior change. In S. A. Shumaker & E. B. Schron (Eds.), *The handbook of health behavior change* (pp. 59–84). New York: Springer.

Prochaska, J. O., & Norcross, J. C. (1994). *Systems of psychotherapy: A transtheoretical analysis* (3rd ed.). Pacific Grove, CA: Brooks/Cole.

Prochaska, J. O., & Norcross, J. C. (1999). *Systems of psychotherapy: A transtheoretical analysis* (4th ed.). Pacific Grove, CA: Brooks/Cole.

Prochaska, J. O., Velicer, W. F., DiClemente, C. C., & Fava, J. (1988). Measuring processes of change: Applications to the cessation of smoking. *Journal of Consulting and Clinical Psychology, 56,* 520–528.

Prochaska, J. O., Velicer, W. F., Guadagnoli, E., Rossi, J. S., & DiClemente, C. C. (1991). Patterns of change: Dynamic typology applied to smoking cessation. *Multivariate Behavioral Research, 26,* 83–107.

Prochaska, J. O., Velicer, W. F., Rossi, J. S., Goldstein, M. G., Marcus, B. H., Rakowski, W., Fiore, C., Harlow, L. L., Redding, C. A., Rosenbloom, D., & Rossi, S. R. (1994). Stages of change and decisional balance for twelve problem behaviors. *Health Psychology, 13,* 39–46.

Project MATCH Research Group. (1997a). Matching alcoholism treatments to client heterogeneity: Project MATCH posttreatment drinking outcomes. *Journal of Studies on Alcohol, 58,* 7–29.

Project MATCH Research Group. (1997b). Project MATCH secondary a priori hypotheses. *Addiction, 92,* 1671–1698.

Project MATCH Research Group. (1998a). Matching alcoholism treatments to client heterogeneity: Project MATCH three year drinking outcomes. *Alcoholism: Clinical and Experimental Research, 22,* 1300–1311.

Project MATCH Research Group. (1998b). Therapist effects in three treatments for alcohol problems. *Psychotherapy Research, 8,* 455–474.

RachBeisel, J., Scott, J., & Dixon, L. (1999). Co-occurring severe mental illness and substance use disorders: A review of recent research. *Psychiatric Services, 50,* 1427–1434.

Ramlow, B. E., White, A. L., Watson, M. A., & Leukefeld, C. G. (1997). The needs of women with substance use problems: An expanded vision for treatment. *Substance Use and Misuse, 32,* 1395–1404.

Randall, C. L., Roberts, J. S., Del Boca, F. K., Carroll, K. M., Connors, G. J., & Mattson, M. E. (1999). Telescoping of landmark events associated with drinking: A gender comparison. *Journal of Studies on Alcohol, 60,* 252–260.

Regier, D. A., Farmer, M. E., Rae, O. S., Locke, B. Z., Keith, S. J., Judd, L. L., & Goodwin, F. K. (1990). Comorbidity of mental disorders with alcohol and other drug abuse. *Journal of the American Medical Association, 264,* 2511–2518.

Rice, D. P., Kelman, S., Miller, L. S., & Dunmeyer, S. (1990). *The economic costs of alcohol and drug abuse and mental illness: 1985.* San Francisco: Institute for Health and Aging.

Ries, R. (1993). Clinical treatment matching models for dually diagnosed patients. *Psychiatric Clinics of North America, 16,* 167–175.

Ries, R. (1994). *Assessment and treatment of patients with coexisting mental illness and alcohol and other drug abuse* (Treatment Improvement Protocol No. 9). Rockville, MD: Center for Substance Abuse Treatment.

Rinaldi, R. C., Steindler, E. M., Wilford, B. B., & Goodwin, D. (1988). Clarification and standardization of substance abuse terminology. *Journal of the American Medical Association, 259,* 555–557.

Roberts, K. S., & Brent, E. E. (1982). Physician utilization and illness patterns in families of alcoholics. *Journal of Studies on Alcohol, 43,* 119–128.

Rogers, R. L., & McMillin, C. S. (1989). *The healing bond: Treating addictions in groups.* New York: Norton.

Rollnick, S., & Heather, N. (1982). The application of Bandura's self-efficacy theory to abstinence-oriented alcoholism treatment. *Addictive Behaviors, 7,* 243–250.

Rollnick, S., Heather, N., Gold, R., & Hall, W. (1992). Development of a short "readiness to change" questionnaire for use in brief, opportunistic interventions among excessive drinkers. *British Journal on Addictions, 87,* 743–754.

Rollnick, S., Mason, P., & Butler, C. (1999) *Health behavior change.* London: Churchill Livingstone.

Room, R. (1989). The U.S. general population's experiences of responding to alcohol problems. *British Journal of Addiction, 84,* 1291–1304.

Rosen, T. J., & Shipley, R. H. (1983). A stage analysis of self-initiated smoking reductions. *Addictive Behaviors, 8,* 263–272.

Rosengren, D., Friese, L., Brennen, S., Donovan, D., & Sloan, K. (1996). *Project START: Treatment interventions.* Unpublished manuscript, Alcohol and Drug Abuse Institute, University of Washington, Seattle.

Ross, H. E., Glaser, F. B., & Germanson, T. (1988). The prevalence of psychiatric disorders in patients with alcohol and other drug problems. *Archives of General Psychiatry, 45,* 1023–1031.

Rotgers, F., Keller, D. S., & Morgenstern, J. (1996). *Treating substance abuse: Theory and technique.* New York: Guilford Press.

Roth, A., & Fonagy, P. (1996). Alcohol dependency and abuse. In A. Roth & P. Fonagy (Eds.), *What works for whom?: A critical review of psychotherapy research* (pp. 216–233). New York: Guilford Press.

Rothfleisch, J. (1997). *Assessing different measures of stages of change with cocaine dependent clients.* Doctoral dissertation, University of Houston.

Rounsaville, B. J. (1986). Clinical implications of relapse research. In F. M. Tims & C. G. Leukefeld (Eds.), *Relapse and recovery in drug abuse* (pp. 172–184). Rockville, MD: National Institute on Drug Abuse.

Rounsaville, B. J., & Carroll, K. M. (1997). Individual psychotherapy. In J. H. Lowinson, P. Ruiz, R. B. Millman, & J. G. Langrod (Eds.), *Substance abuse: A comprehensive textbook* (3rd ed., pp 430–439). Baltimore: Williams & Wilkins.

Rugel, R. P. (1991). Addictions treatment in groups: A review of therapeutic factors. *Small Group Research, 22,* 475–491.

Ryan, R. M., Plant, R. W., & O'Malley, S. (1995). Initial motivations for alcohol treatment: Relations with patient characteristics, treatment involvement, and dropout. *Addictive Behaviors, 20,* 279–297.

Rychtarik, R. G. (1990). Alcohol-related coping skills in spouses of alcoholics: Assessment and implications for treatment. In R. L. Collins, K. E. Leonard, & J. S. Searles (Eds.), *Alcohol and the family: Research and clinical perspectives* (pp. 356–379). New York: Guilford Press.

Rychtarik, R. G., Koutsky, J. R., & Miller, W. R. (1998). Profiles of the Alcohol Use Inventory: A large sample cluster analysis conducted with split-sample replication rules. *Psychological Assessment, 10,* 107–119.

Rychtarik, R. G., Koutsky, J. R., & Miller, W. R. (1999). Profiles of the Alcohol Use Inventory: Correction to Rychtarik, Koutsky, and Miller (1998). *Psychological Assessment, 11,* 396–402.

Rychtarik, R. G., Prue, D. M., Rapp, S. R., & King, A. C. (1992). Self-efficacy, aftercare and relapse in a treatment program for alcoholics. *Journal of Studies on Alcohol, 53,* 435–440.

Salloum, I. M., Moss, H. W., Daley, D. C. (1991). Substance abuse and schizophrenia: Impediments to optimal care. *American Journal of Drug and Alcohol Abuse, 17,* 321–336.

Salloum, I. M., Moss, H. B., Daley, D. C., Cornelius, J. R., Kirisci, L., & Al-Maalouf, M. (1998). Drug use problem awareness and treatment readiness in dual-diagnosis patients. *American Journal on Addictions, 7,* 35–42.

Sanchez-Craig, M., Annis, H. M., Bornet, A. R., & MacDonald, K. R. (1984). Random assignment to abstinence and controlled drinking: Evaluation of a cognitive behavioral program for problem drinkers. *Journal of Consulting and Clinical Psychology, 52,* 390–403.

Sandahl, C., Linberg, S., & Ronnberg, S. (1990). Efficacy expectations among alcohol-dependent patients: A Swedish version of the Situational Confidence Questionnaire. *Alcohol and Alcoholism, 25,* 67–73.

Sandler, J., Holder, A., & Dare, C. (1970). Basic psychoanalytic concepts: V. Resistance. *British Journal of Psychiatry, 117,* 215–221.

Saunders, B., Baily, S., Phillips, M., & Allsop, S. (1993). Women with alcohol problems: Do they relapse for reasons different to their male counterparts? *Addiction, 88,* 1413–1422.

Saunders, B., Wilkinson, C., & Allsop, S. (1991). Motivational intervention with heroin users attending a methadone clinic. In W. R. Miller & S. Rollnick, *Motivational interviewing: Preparing people to change addictive behavior* (pp. 279–292). New York: Guilford Press.

Saunders, J. B., Aasland, O. G., Babor, T. F., de la Fuente, J. R., & Grant, M. (1993). Development of the Alcohol Use Disorders Identification Test (AUDIT): WHO collaborative project on early detection of persons with harmful alcohol consumption—II. *Addiction, 88,* 791–804.

Schmidt, L., & Weisner, C. (1995). The emergence of problem-drinking women as a special population in need of treatment. In M. Galanter (Ed.), *Recent advances in alcoholism: Vol. 12. Alcoholism and women* (pp. 309–334). New York: Plenum Press.

Schober, R., & Annis, H. M. (1996). Barriers to help-seeking for change in drinking: A gender-focused review of the literature. *Addictive Behaviors, 21,* 81–92.

Schonfeld, L., Peters, R., & Dolente, A. (1993). *SARA. Substance Abuse Relapse Assessment: Professional manual.* Odessa, FL: Psychological Assessment Resources, Inc.

Schonfeld, L., Rohrer, G. E., Dupree, L. W., & Thomas, M. (1989). Antecedents of relapse and recent substance use. *Community Mental Health Journal, 25,* 245–249.

Schuckit, M. A., Anthenelli, R. M., Bucholz, K. K., Hesselbrock, V. M., & Tipp, J. (1995). The time course of development of alcohol-related problems in men and women. *Journal of Studies on Alcohol, 56,* 218–225.

Schuckit, M. A., Daeppen, J. B., Tipp, J. E., Hesselbrock, M., & Bucholz, K. K. (1998). The clinical course of alcohol-related problems in alcohol dependent and nonalcohol dependent drinking women and men. *Journal of Studies on Alcohol, 59,* 581–590.

Schulz, J. E., & Chappel, J. N. (1998). Twelve step programs. In A. W. Graham, T. K. Schultz, & B. B. Wilford (Eds.), *Principles of addiction medicine* (pp. 693–705). Chevy Chase, MD: American Society of Addiction Medicine.

Schwartz, R. H. (1988). Screening for drug use in adolescents: The other side of the coin. *Journal of Pediatrics, 112,* 328.

Selzer, M. L. (1971). The Michigan Alcoholism Screening Test: The quest for a new diagnostic instrument. *American Journal of Psychiatry, 127,* 1653–1658.

Selzer, M. L., Vinokur, A., & van Rooijen, L. (1975). A self-administered short Michigan Alcoholism Screening Test (SMAST). *Journal of Studies on Alcohol, 36,* 117–126.

Shaffer, H. J. (1992). The psychology of stage change: The transition from addiction to recovery. In J. H. Lowison, P. Ruiz, R. B. Millman, & J. G. Langrod (Eds.), *Substance abuse: A comprehensive textbook* (2nd ed., pp. 100–105). Baltimore: Williams & Wilkins.

Sher, K. J. (1997). Psychological characteristics of children of alcoholics. *Alcohol Health and Research World, 21,* 247–254.

Sheridan, M. J. (1995). A proposed intergenerational model of substance abuse, family functioning, and abuse/neglect. *Child Abuse and Neglect, 19,* 519–530.

Shiffman, S. (1989). Conceptual issues in the study of relapse. In M. Gossop (Ed.), *Relapse and addictive behavior* (pp. 149–179). London: Tavistock/Routledge.

Siegal, H. A., Fisher, J. H., Rapp, R. C., Wagner, J. H., Forney, M. A., & Callejo, V. (1995). Presenting problems of substance abusers in treatment: Implications for service delivery and attrition. *American Journal on Drug and Alcohol Abuse, 21,* 17–26.

Silverman, K., Chutuape, M. A. D., Bigelow, G. E., & Stitzer, M. L. (1996). Voucher-based reinforcement of attendance by unemployed methadone patients in a job skills training program. *Drug and Alcohol Dependence, 41,* 197–207.

Silverman, K., Wong, C. J., Umbricht-Schneiter, A., Montoya, I. D., Schuster, C. R., & Preston, K. L. (1998). Broad beneficial effects of cocaine abstinence reinforcement among methadone patients. *Journal of Consulting and Clinical Psychology, 66,* 811–824.

Simpson, D. D., & Joe, G. W. (1993). Motivation as a predictor of early drop out from drug abuse treatment. *Psychotherapy, 30,* 357–368.

Simpson, D. D., Joe, G. W., Rowan-Szal, G., & Greener, J. (1995). Client engagement and change during drug abuse treatment. *Journal of Substance Abuse, 7,* 117–134.

Sisson, R. W., & Azrin, N. H. (1993). Community reinforcement training for families: A method to get alcoholics into treatment. In T. J. O'Farrell (Ed.), *Treating alcohol problems: Marital and family interventions* (pp. 34–53). New York: Guilford Press.

Sitharthan, T., & Kavanagh, D. J. (1991). Role of self-efficacy in predicting outcomes from a programme for controlled drinking. *Drug and Alcohol Dependence, 27,* 87–94.

Skinner, H. A. (1982). The Drug Abuse Screening Test. *Addictive Behaviors, 7,* 363–371.

Skinner, H. A., & Allen, B. A. (1983). Differential assessment of alcoholism: Evaluation of the Alcohol Use Inventory. *Journal of Studies on Alcohol, 44,* 852–862.

Smith, K. J., Subich, L. M., & Kalodner, C. (1995). The transtheoretical model's stages and processes of change and their relation to premature termination. *Journal of Counseling Psychology, 42,* 34–39.

Smith, L. (1992). Help seeking in alcohol-dependent females. *Alcohol and Alcoholism, 27,* 3–9.

Smyth, N. J. (1996). Motivating persons with dual disorders: A stage approach. *Families in Society, 77,* 605–614.

Snow, M., Prochaska, J., & Rossi, J. (1994). Processes of change in Alcoholics Anonymous: Maintenance factors in long-term sobriety. *Journal of Studies on Alcohol, 55*, 362–371.

Sobell, L. C., Cunningham, J. A., Sobell, M. B., & Toneatto, T. (1993). A life-span perspective on natural recovery (self-change) from alcohol problems. In J. S. Baer, G. A. Marlatt, & R. J. McMahon (Eds.), *Addictive behaviors across the life span* (pp. 34–66). Newbury Park, CA: Sage Publications.

Sobell, L. C., Maisto, S. A., Sobell, M. B., & Cooper, A. M. (1979). Reliability of alcohol abusers' self-reports of drinking behavior. *Behaviour Research and Therapy, 17*, 157–160.

Sobell, L. C., & Sobell, M. B. (1992). Timeline follow-back: A technique for assessing self-reported alcohol consumption. In R. Litten & J. Allen (Eds.), *Measuring alcohol consumption* (pp. 41–72). Totowa, NJ: Humana Press.

Sobell, L. C., & Sobell, M. B. (1996). *Alcohol Timeline Followback (TLFB) users' manual.* Toronto, Canada: Addiction Research Foundation.

Sobell, L. C., Sobell, M. B., & Nirenberg, T. D. (1982). Differential treatment planning for alcohol abusers. In E. M. Pattison & E. Kaufman (Eds.), *Encyclopedic handbook of alcoholism* (pp. 1140–1151). New York: Gardner Press.

Sobell, L. C., Sobell, M. B., & Nirenberg, T. D. (1988). Behavioral assessment and treatment planning with alcohol and drug abusers: A review with an emphasis on clinical application. *Clinical Psychology Review, 8*, 19–54.

Sobell, L. C., Sobell, M. B., Toneatto, T., & Leo, G. I. (1993). What triggers the resolution of alcohol problems without treatment? *Alcoholism: Clinical and Experimental Research, 17*, 217–224.

Sobell, L. C., Toneatto, T., & Sobell, M. B. (1994). Behavioral assessment and treatment planning for alcohol, tobacco, and other drug problems: Current status with an emphasis on clinical applications. *Behavior Therapy, 25*, 533–580.

Sobell, M. B., Bogardis, J., Schuller, R., Leo, G. I., & Sobell, L. C. (1989). Is self-monitoring of alcohol consumption reactive? *Behavioral Assessment, 11*, 447–458.

Sobell, M. B., & Sobell, L. C. (1981). Functional analysis of alcohol problems. In C. K. Prokop and L. A. Bradley (Eds.), *Medical psychology: Contributions to behavioral medicine* (pp. 81–90). New York: Academic Press.

Sobell, M. B., & Sobell, L. C. (1993). *Problem drinkers: Guided self-change treatment.* New York: Guilford Press.

Solomon, K. E., & Annis, H. M. (1990). Outcome and efficacy expectancy in the prediction of posttreatment drinking behaviour. *British Journal of Addiction, 85*, 659–665.

Solomon, R. L. (1980). The opponent-process theory of acquired motivation: The costs of pleasure and the benefits of pain. *American Psychologist, 35*, 691–712.

Spinks, S. H., & Birchler, G. R. (1982). Behavioral-systems marital therapy: Dealing with resistance. *Family Process, 21*, 169–185.

Stanislav, S. W., Sommi, R. W., & Watson, W. A. (1992). A longitudinal analysis of factors associated with morbidity in cocaine abusers with psychiatric illness. *Pharmacotherapy, 12*, 114–118.

Stanton, M. D. (1997). The role of family and significant others in the engagement and retention of drug-dependent individuals. In L. S. Onken, J. D. Blaine, & F. J. Boren (Eds.), *Beyond the therapeutic alliance: Keeping the drug dependent individual in treatment* (pp. 157–180). Rockville, MD: National Institute on Drug Abuse.

Stasiewicz, P. R., Bradizza, C. M., & Maisto, S. A. (1997). Alcohol problem resolution in the severely mentally ill: A preliminary investigation. *Journal of Substance Abuse, 9,* 209–222.

Stasiewicz, P. R., Carey, K. B., Bradizza, C. M., & Maisto, S. A. (1996). Behavioral assessment of substance abuse with co-occurring psychiatric disorder. *Cognitive and Behavioral Practice, 3,* 91–105.

Steinhausen, H. C. (1995). Children of alcoholic parents: A review. *European Child and Adolescent Psychiatry, 4,* 419–432.

Stinchfield, R., Owen, P. L., & Winters, K. C. (1994). Group therapy for substance abuse: A review of the empirical evidence. In A. Fuhriman & G. M. Burlinggame (Eds.), *Handbook of group psychotherapy: An empirical and clinical synthesis* (pp. 458–488). New York: Wiley.

Stotts, A., DiClemente, C. C., Carbonari, J. P., & Mullen, P. (1996). Pregnancy smoking cessation: A case of mistaken identity. *Addictive Behaviors, 21,* 459–471.

Stotts, A. L., DiClemente, C. C., Carbonari, J. P., & Mullen, P. D. (2000). Postpartum return to smoking: Staging a "suspended" behavior. *Health Psychology, 19,* 324–332.

Straussner, S. L. A. (1997). Group treatment with substance abusing clients: A model of treatment during the early phases of outpatient group therapy. *Journal of Chemical Dependency Treatment, 7,* 67–80.

Sullivan, W. P. (1994). Case management and community-based treatment of women with substance abuse problems. *Journal of Case Management, 3,* 158–161.

Sutton, S. (1996). Can "stage of change" provide guidance in treatment of addiction? A critical examination of Prochaska & DiClemente's model. In G. Edwards & C. Dare (Eds.), *Psychotherapy, psychological treatments and the addictions.* New York: Cambridge University Press.

Swanson, A. J., Pantalon, M. V., & Cohen, K. R. (1999). Motivational interviewing and treatment adherence among psychiatric and dually diagnosed patients. *Journal of Nervous and Mental Disease, 187,* 630–635.

Swenson, W. M., & Morse, R. M. (1975). The use of a Self-Administered Alcoholism Screening Test (SAAST) in a medical center. *Mayo Clinic Proceedings, 50,* 204–208.

Szuster, R. R., Rich, L. L., Chung, A., & Bisconer, S. W. (1996). Treatment retention in women's residential chemical dependency treatment: The effect of admission with children. *Substance Use and Misuse, 31,* 1001–1013.

Thom, B. (1987). Sex differences in help-seeking for alcohol problems: Entry into treatment. *British Journal of Addiction, 82,* 989–997.

Thomas, E. J. (1994). The spouse as a positive rehabilitative influence in reaching the uncooperative alcohol abuser. In D. K. Granvold (Ed.), *Cognitive and behavioral treatment: Methods and applications* (pp. 159–173). Pacific Grove, CA: Brooks/Cole.

Thomas, E. J., & Ager, R. D. (1993). Unilateral family therapy with spouses of uncooperative alcohol abusers. In T. J. O'Farrell (Ed.), *Treating alcohol problems: Marital and family interventions* (pp. 3–33). New York: Guilford Press.

Thomas, E. J., & Santa, C. A. (1982). Unilateral family therapy for alcohol abuse: A working conception. *American Journal of Family Therapy, 10,* 49–58.

Thomas, E. J., Santa, C., Bronson, D., & Oyserman, D. (1987). Unilateral family therapy with the spouses of alcoholics. *Journal of Social Service Research, 10,* 145–162.

Thomas, E. J., Yoshioka, M., & Ager, R. D. (1996). Spouse enabling of alcohol abuse: Conception, assessment, and modification. *Journal of Substance Abuse, 8,* 61–80.

Thoreson, R. W., & Budd, F. C. (1987). Self-help groups and other group procedures for treating alcohol problems. In W. M. Cox (Ed.), *Treatment and prevention of alcohol problems: A resource manual* (pp. 157–181). Orlando, FL: Academic Press.

Tiffany, S. T. (1990). A cognitive model of drug urges and drug-use behavior: Role of automatic and nonautomatic processes. *Psychological Review, 97,* 147–168.

Tiffany, S. T. (1992). A critique of contemporary urge and craving research: Methodological, psychometric, and theoretical issues. *Advances in Behaviour Research and Therapy, 14,* 123–139.

Tonigan, J. S., & Hiller-Sturmhofel, S. (1994). Alcoholics Anonymous: Who benefits? *Alcohol Health and Research World, 18,* 308–310.

Tonigan, J. S., Miller, W. R., & Brown, J. M. (1997). The reliability of Form 90: An instrument for assessing alcohol treatment outcome. *Journal of Studies on Alcohol, 58,* 358–364.

Tsoh, J. (1995). *Stages of change, drop-outs and outcome in substance abuse treatment.* Doctoral dissertation, University of Rhode Island, Kingston.

Tucker, J. A., Vuchinich, R. E., & Pukish, M. M. (1995). Molar environmental contexts surrounding recovery from alcohol problems by treated and untreated problem drinkers. *Experimental and Clinical Psychopharmacology, 3,* 195–204.

Turkat, I. D., & Meyer, V. (1982). The behavior-analytic approach. In P. L. Wachtel (Ed.), *Resistance: Psychodynamic and behavioral approaches* (pp. 157–184). New York: Plenum Press.

U. S. Department of Health and Human Services. (1998). *Preliminary findings from the 1997 National Household Survey on Drug Abuse.* Washington, DC: Substance Abuse and Mental Health Services Administration.

Vaillant, G. E. (1977). *Adaptation to life.* Boston: Little, Brown.

Vaillant, G. E. (1995). *The natural history of alcoholism revisited.* Cambridge, MA: Harvard University Press.

van Bilsen, H. P., & van Emst, A. J. (1986). Heroin addiction and motivational milieu therapy. *International Journal of the Addictions, 21,* 707–713.

Vannicelli, M. (1982). Group psychotherapy with alcoholics: Special techniques. *Journal of Studies on Alcohol, 43,* 17–37.

Vannicelli, M. (1992). *Removing the roadblocks: Group psychotherapy with substance abusers and family members.* New York: Guilford Press.

Velasquez, M. M., Carbonari, J. P., & DiClemente, C. C. (1999). Psychiatric severity and behavior change in alcoholism: The relation of the transtheoretical model variables to psychiatric distress in dually diagnosed patients. *Addictive Behaviors, 24,* 481–496.

Velasquez, M. M., Maurer, G., Crouch, C., & DiClemente, C. C. (2001). *Group treatment for substance abuse: A stages-of-change therapy manual.* New York: Guilford Press.

Velicer, W. F., Prochaska, J. O., Bellis, J. M., DiClemente, C. C., Rossi, J. S., Fava, J. L., & Steiger, J. H. (1993). An expert system intervention for smoking cessation. *Addictive Behaviors, 18,* 269–290.

Vinogradov, S., & Yalom, I. D. (1989). *A concise guide to group psychotherapy.* Washington, DC: American Psychiatric Press.

Wallace, B. B. (1989). Psychological and environmental determinants of relapse in crack cocaine smokers. *Journal of Substance Abuse Treatment, 6,* 95–106.

Wanberg, K. W., Horn, J. L., & Foster, F. M. (1977). A differential assessment model of alcoholism: The scales of the Alcohol Use Inventory. *Journal of Studies on Alcohol, 38,* 512–543.

Washton, A. M. (1987). Outpatient treatment techniques. In A. M. Washton & M. S. Gold (Eds.), *Cocaine: A clinician's handbook* (pp. 106–117). New York: Guilford Press.

Washton, A. M. (1988). Preventing relapse to cocaine. *Journal of Clinical Psychiatry*, *49*(Suppl.), 34–38.

Washton, A. M. (1992). Structured outpatient group therapy with alcohol and substance abusers. In J. H. Lowinson, P. Ruiz, R. B. Millman, & J. G. Langrod (Eds.), *Substance abuse: A comprehensive textbook* (pp. 508–519). Baltimore: Williams & Wilkins.

Watson, R. R., Mohs, M. E., Eskelson, C., Sampliner, E., & Hartmann, B. (1986). Identification of alcohol abuse and alcoholism with biological parameters. *Alcoholism: Clinical and Experimental Research*, *10*, 364–385.

Weiss, R. D., & Collins, D. A. (1992). Substance abuse and psychiatric illness: The dually diagnosed patient. *American Journal on Addictions*, *1*, 93–99.

Weissberg, J. H., & Levay, A. N. (1981). The role of resistance in sex therapy. *Journal of Sex and Marital Therapy*, *7*, 125–130.

Werch, C. E., & DiClemente, C. C. (1994). A multi-component stage model for matching drug prevention strategies and messages to youth stage of use. *Health Education Research: Theory and Practice*, *9*, 37–46.

Whitfield, C. L. (1989). Co-dependence: Our most common addiction: Some physical, mental, emotional and spiritual perspectives. *Alcoholism Treatment Quarterly*, *6*, 19–36.

Wholey, D. (1984). *The courage to change*. New York: Warner Books.

Wickizer, T., Maynard, C., Artherly, A., Frederick, M., Koepsell, T., Krupski, A., & Stark, K. (1994). Completion rates of clients discharged from drug and alcohol treatment programs in Washington state. *American Journal of Public Health*, *84*, 215–221.

Wilkinson, D. A., & LeBreton, S. (1986). Early indications of treatment outcome in multiple drug users. In W. R. Miller & N. Heather (Eds.), *Treating addictive behaviors* (pp. 239–261). New York: Plenum Press.

Will, D. (1983). Some techniques for working with resistant families of adolescents. *Journal of Adolescence*, *6*, 13–26.

Willoughby, F. W., & Edens, J. F. (1996). Construct validity and predictive utility of the stages of change scale for alcoholics. *Journal of Substance Abuse*, *8*, 275–291.

Wilsnack, S. C. (1991). Barriers to treatment for alcoholic women. *Addiction and Recovery*, *11*, 10–12.

Wise, R. A. (1988). The neurobiology of craving: Implications for the understanding and treatment of addiction. *Journal of Abnormal Psychology*, *97*, 118–132.

Yalom, I. (1995). *The theory and practice of group psychotherapy* (4th ed.). New York: Basic Books.

Yoshioka, M. R., Thomas, E. J., & Ager, R. D. (1992). Nagging and other drinking control efforts of spouses and uncooperative alcohol abusers: Assessment and modification. *Journal of Substance Abuse*, *4*, 309–318.

Yu, M. M., & Watkins, T. (1996). Group counseling with DUI offenders: A model using client anger to enhance group cohesion and movement. *Alcoholism Treatment Quarterly*, *14*, 47–57.

Zywiak, W. H., Connors, G. J., Maisto, S. A., & Westerberg, V. S. (1996). Relapse research and the Reasons for Drinking Questionnaire: A factor analysis of Marlatt's taxonomy. *Addiction*, *91*(Suppl.), 121–130.

INDEX